PRAISE FOR *TRANSFORMATIVE HEALTHCARE*

If you want clear, rational insights into how to transform healthcare, Kuhlman and Peach have encapsulated **an intuitively compelling, foundational, flexible framework that healthcare leaders and providers alike can implement.**
> **James L. Gulley**, MD, PhD, FACP
> Director, Medical Oncology Service, Center for Cancer Research,
> National Cancer Institute, National Institutes of Health

Whether you are a health system leader, or a physician discouraged with the state of healthcare, this book is for you. *Transformative Healthcare: A Physician-Led Prescription to Save Thousands of Lives and Millions of Dollars* is just that: a way out of the healthcare delivery system quagmire we are currently experiencing. I write this as a physician who has seen multiple ideas come and go with limited effect and too many electronic medical record chokeholds. It was exciting to experience the positive changes described in this book as I cared for my patients. **This is a breath of fresh air. It respects the motives and experiences of the frontline worker and is a blueprint to harness this energy.**
> **Kathleen Clem**, MD, FACEP
> Professor, Emergency Medicine,
> Geisel School of Medicine at Dartmouth

Transformative Healthcare **is a remarkable combination of breakthrough thinking and common sense, full of powerful ideas for achievable healthcare innovation.** How refreshing it is to hear a compelling, evidence-based case for truly putting the doctor-patient relationship at the center of healthcare, as opposed to "lean" business models, compliance checklists, or ever more technology analyzing ever more data. Like Dr. Kuhlman's experience in the White House, my formative years in the Emergency Department taught me to pay close attention to the human being in front of me, and to synthesize both data and good judgment to arrive at the right course of treatment, an approach that—not incidentally—saves both lives and money. This book is chockfull of "aha!" stories and actionable insights for any healthcare organization, even amid multiple health system crises, and even for small teams with a small budget for innovation. **In short, this is the freshest, most resonant, and compelling thinking I have encountered in my career on how to improve America's healthcare system.**

    James A. D'Orta, MD, FACEP
    Trustee, Board of Directors, MedStar Health
    Assistant Clinical Professor,
    Georgetown University School of Medicine

***Transformative Healthcare* is a timely and much needed book.** As a result of a global pandemic, the safety and integrity of our healthcare delivery systems are on the minds of most citizens. Our industry is inherently complex and is one that is difficult to create significant positive change for the better over time. What gets lost in this complexity, at times, is the importance of relationships. The patient-physician relationship remains the dominant relationship that drives the delivery of care, but there are numerous other relationship types that are critically important as well. The authors offer strong insights on the necessary focus needed toward relationships in healthcare delivery and provide helpful approaches on how to improve care while simultaneously reducing the complexity and inefficiencies found in today's environment of clinical care. **If you truly want to get to patient-centered care, then this is a must-read book.**

>**Peter Angood**, MD
>President & Chief Executive Officer
>American Association for Physician Leadership (AAPL)
>Washington, DC and Tampa, FL
>Author, *All Physicians Are Leaders*

Jeffrey Kuhlman and Daniel Peach have made an extremely valuable contribution to inform our thinking about fundamental change and improvement in the American healthcare system. In *Transformative Healthcare*, these two experts bring their broad expertise to bear. **They have provided a practical, systematic, and well-thought-out approach to the healthcare changes that are so desperately needed.**

>**Michael Leonard**, MD
>Founding Partner, Safe & Reliable Healthcare LLC

There are literally hundreds of books written about 'transforming' healthcare in the United States which today is more of an 'enterprise' (not a system) that has been uniquely designed to cost a lot of money while not delivering on the promise of improving the quality of care. **In their excellent book, *Transformative Healthcare*, Jeff Kuhlman and Daniel Peach describe a proven, common-sense approach to real transformation in delivering quality care at lower cost** by shifting from the current-day rigidity of evidence-based medicine to the flexibility of practice-based evidence in providing care truly focused on the patient. They describe this as 'synthetical thinking' where the physician absorbs subjective and objective feedback from all sources—especially by listening to and examining the patient—then adapting the care plan for that patient. In short, they are describing the critical thinking that is inherent to training in family medicine and primary care; not surprising given that Jeff Kuhlman is a family physician.

I especially appreciate their caution that the use of technology and data should complement—and not drive—the delivery of healthcare to patients as is so often the case today. And with the evolving use of AI in healthcare, this caution is well taken. **The primacy of the patient-physician relationship over time is critical, as is their recognition of the importance of practice experience, personal and demonstrated expertise, and observation in delivering quality patient care.** This is especially true given that most patients, most of the time, present with a set of undifferentiated signs and symptoms – situations where 'patient-first algorithms' can be powerful tools to assure quality and lower overall costs yet must have the needed flexibility for expected patient variability. Their experience at AdventHealth critically demonstrates that such "patient-first algorithms" in transforming care must be derived from the physicians and clinicians providing the daily frontline medical care in order to achieve and sustain such transformation.

This is a book I would highly recommend to anyone seriously looking to improve the quality and cost of healthcare in the US today. I only wish they had provided some examples of such transformation and improvement in the primary care ambulatory environment as most healthcare happens in this environment, not the hospital, and the evidence clearly shows that foundational primary care can itself be "transformational." Perhaps a subsequent book by Kuhlman and Peach may describe such learnings and success.

Douglas E. Henley, MD, FAAFP
Executive Vice President/CEO Emeritus
American Academy of Family Physicians

From Navy flight surgeon to Physician to the President of the United States to hospital executive, Dr. Jeff Kuhlman has spent his entire career taking care of patients. With passion and purpose, Dr. Kuhlman describes how his experiences from patient bedside to hospital boardroom have enabled him to develop practical and effective ways to improve patient care in America. **This is a must-read for all healthcare professionals who strive to transform healthcare.**

    E. Connie Mariano, MD, FACP
    Rear Admiral, U. S. Navy (retired)
    Former White House Doctor and Physician to the President
    President, Center for Executive Medicine, Scottsdale, AZ
    Author, *The White House Doctor: My Patients Were Presidents*

This book is a must-read for all healthcare providers, administrators, and essentially anyone who may ever need medical care. It is an extremely interesting guide to how medicine should be practiced optimizing patient outcomes and limiting the cost of healthcare. The authors are genuine in their desire to transform healthcare emphasizing the need for the patient-physician relationship to take priority and be served rather than hindered by modern technology and a tedious electronic medical record. **For those experienced in the practice of medicine, the book is a wonderful reminder of why we entered the field in the first place.** For those just getting started, it educates in a way that we hope medicine is being taught in the world today.

Ultimately for those requiring medical assistance it gives hope that in their time of need the thing they will require most, a strong caring relationship with their providers, will be there assisted by the most modern medical technology. The authors emphasize the importance of trusting experience in addition to the data. They offer their own exciting and unique lifetime experiences which are captivating and used in such a way that allows all readers, including those with no medical knowledge, the ability to understand the obstacles and relate to their transformative methods that have led to enormous cost savings and significantly improved outcomes at their institution. **Simply stated, the book is a reminder that caring relationships, experience, and the drive and ability to always do the right thing for patients under any circumstances must take priority,** be optimized and not hindered by modern technology, and remain permanently at the core of healthcare in our future.

    Louis R Pizano, MD, MBA, FACS
    Professor of Surgery and Anesthesiology
    Chief, Division of Burns
    Director, Trauma and Surgical Critical Care Fellowship Program
    DeWitt Daughtry Family Department of Surgery
    University of Miami Miller School of Medicine

Dr. Jeff Kuhlman's concept of treating each patient as if he or she were the president is powerful. Every clinician feeling the responsibility of caring for a patient as if they were the Leader of the Free World undoubtedly would transform healthcare—as well as every domain of care delivery. Indeed, properly personalizing care leaves no room for relying on unreliable approaches such as the "See something, say something" method for identifying safety problems or reactively handling the risk of injury or death after the fact by effectively using "rearview mirror" management. We can and should do better in the age of digitally assisted care, which makes Dr. Kuhlman's call **especially timely and a critical imperative."**

    Drew Ladner, MA, MBA
    Chairman & CEO of Pascal Metrics
    Former Chief Information Officer, U.S. Department of the Treasury

The authors use their rich and distinctive lifelong journeys navigating diverse healthcare systems to illustrate innovative and timely approaches to healthcare delivery. The chapters powerfully connect the authors' experiences from memory lane with valuable theories that have stood the test of time and that are crucial for today's healthcare managers to understand and be able to apply effectively. This text is an enjoyable, and at times emotional, reading experience that will bring both healthcare professionals and anyone who has engaged with healthcare systems directly or indirectly to a halt to reflect on each one of the well-sequenced and provocatively titled chapters. The authors facilitate the readers' journey by offering "Key Points" and "Reflections" on important concepts such as synthetical thinking clouds, the cost of reactionary healthcare, practice-based evidence, and moonshot innovations. The readings will leave you wondering about topics such as how we know when change is attained, the connections between healthcare and law enforcement, and what similarities doctors share with chefs. As the authors affirm, "the future is now," and we, the readers, are invited to envision and realize our own bold transformational approaches to healthcare.

    Bernardo Ramirez, MD, MBA
        Associate Professor and Director of Global Health Initiatives
        Department of Health Management & Informatics
        College of Community Innovation and Education
        University of Central Florida, Downtown Campus

The genius of Kuhlman and Peach's *Transformative Healthcare* lies in its simplicity of explanation. I found myself shaking my head many times in agreement as I read each chapter. The explanations are tied to everyday common-sense examples that clearly articulate the need for change in healthcare and the way in which that change can be implemented. Again and again, the reader sees the challenge, the depth and breadth of that challenge, and the remarkably elegant solution to each problem. **This is a book for everyone in healthcare, from Allied Health Professionals to providers to administrators.**

>**Jeffrey M Hardin**, MD, MBA, CPE, FACC
>Chief of Cardiology, AdventHealth Hendersonville

Doctors and patients alike agree that the American medical system is horribly broken. Kuhlman and Peach have forged a bold, visionary path which leads us back to the root of medicine: the doctor and the patient. Modern technology, systems, and protocols can be quickly turned to serve the patient first. **If medicine is leaving you frustrated, burned out, and exhausted, now is the time to follow these distinguished healers to the place you wanted to be when you chose medicine. You can start today!**

>**Lewis A. Hofmann**, MD, FAAFP
>Col (ret) USAF, MC, FS
>Former White House Physician

Dr. Kuhlman, during his time at the White House, was in a position that very few doctors in the world were in; he became aware of cutting-edge technologies and the latest medicines that provide the best personalized care in the world . . . for one person! This book is his way of directing the healthcare system and the rest of us towards that goal. I also love the anecdotes in his book, as we've had similar experiences.

>**Rami Farraj**, MD, FRCP, FACP, FRCP (Edin.)
>Private Physician to His Majesty King Abdullah II of Jordan

A must-read for anyone with an interest in the U.S. healthcare system, either as a healthcare provider, hospital administrator, or patient. Drs. Kuhlman and Peach have devised an intuitively simple yet very effective approach to caring for patients that emphasizes the basics of the physician-patient relationship and that underscores how everything we do as part of the healthcare team should logically follow from that relationship. Acknowledging the importance of advances in technology and scientific breakthroughs, the authors argue that the best healthcare involves using these advances as tools in the service of the patient rather than as a replacement for that. This was the approach that Dr. Kuhlman utilized as Physician-in-Chief to the President of the United States and, contrary to conventional wisdom, makes sense not only from a patient care perspective but also as a way of reining in healthcare dollars spent. And rather than dwell on what is wrong with the healthcare "industry," the authors provide specific comments and suggestions on how to improve it. If, indeed, what we do as physicians is to alleviate pain, prevent disability, and postpone death, then **the prescription written by Drs. Kuhlman and Peach is the one likely to heal what ails the U.S. healthcare system.**

> **Bradley A. Connor**, MD, AGA-F, FIDSA, FACP, FRCPS (Glas)
> Clinical Professor of Medicine, Weill Cornell Medical College
> Past President, International Society of Travel Medicine
> Consultant to the Centers for Disease Control and Prevention (CDC) and White House Medical Unit

I don't normally comment on the books I narrate, but *Transformative Healthcare* **made a strong impact on me.** It's remarkable how just one "algorithm" of care saved 1,500 lives in just a few months. We've known for decades that we can count the cost of bureaucracy in "lives lost." **I pray that we do away with unnecessary protocols and processes, and that more hospitals and clinics will commit to the patient-centered care emphasized in this book.**

> **Tim Lundeen**
> Narrator of over 100 audiobooks including
> *Transformative Healthcare*

TRANSFORMATIVE HEALTHCARE

Kelly,
Thank you for your leadership!

Jeffrey Kullman

JEFFREY KUHLMAN, MD, MPH
and
DANIEL J. PEACH
with
ROBERT STEPHENS

Advent
Health
Press

TRANSFORMATIVE HEALTHCARE

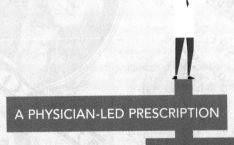

A PHYSICIAN-LED PRESCRIPTION
TO SAVE THOUSANDS OF LIVES
AND MILLIONS OF DOLLARS

AdventHealth

Transformative Healthcare
Copyright © MMXXI Jeffrey Kuhlman, MD, & Daniel J. Peach
Published by AdventHealth Press
605 Montgomery Road, Altamonte Springs, Florida 32714

EXTENDING *the* HEALING MINISTRY *of* CHRIST

Editor-in-Chief	Todd Chobotar
Managing Editor	Denise Rougeux-Putt
Collaborative Writer	Robert Stephens
Internal Peer Reviewers	Joyce Kerpchar, PA-C, MBA, CPPS
	Piotr Kulach, PhD
External Peer Reviewers	Allan Frankel, MD
	Lou Pizano, MD, FACS
Copy Editor	Pam Nordberg
Promotion	Caryn McCleskey
Production	Lillian Boyd
Photography	Spencer Freeman
Cover Design	John Lucas
Interior Design	Frank Gutbrod
Cartoon Illustrator	Dana Boyd

PUBLISHER'S NOTE: This book is not intended to replace a one-on-one relationship with a qualified healthcare professional but as a sharing of knowledge and information from the research and experience of the authors. You are advised and encouraged to consult with your healthcare professional in all matters relating to your health and the health of your family. The publisher and authors disclaim any liability arising directly or indirectly from the use of this book.

AUTHOR'S NOTE: This book contains many case histories and patient stories. In order to preserve the privacy of some of the people involved, we have disguised names, appearances, and aspects of their personal stories so they are not identifiable. Patient stories may also include composite characters.

NOT TO BE REPRODUCED
No portion of this book may be reproduced, stored in a retrieval system, or transmitted in any form or by any means—electronic, mechanical, photocopy, recording, or any other—except for brief quotations in printed reviews, without the prior written permission of the publisher. All rights reserved.

For special orders, events, or other information, please contact:
AdventHealthPress.com | 407-200-8224

AdventHealth Press is a wholly owned entity of AdventHealth.
Library of Congress Control number: 2021911808
Printed in the United States of America.
PR 14 13 12 11 10 9 8 7 6 5 4 3 2 1
ISBN: 978-1-7342984-9-9 (Print)
ISBN: 978-1-7372507-1-5 EBook)

For other life-changing resources visit:
AdventHealthPress.com
CREATIONLife.com

Dedication

To the women and men on the front line of healthcare

Dr. Jeff Kuhlman is donating author royalties to the

Whole Person Health Education Fund

at AdventHealth Foundation.

To discover how you can make a

meaningful difference, please visit

www.GenerosityHeals.Health

Contents

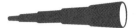

FOREWORD	01
INTRODUCTION *This Is Our Purpose*	05
1. OUR BEDS ARE ON FIRE *So Why Are We Waiting for Someone Else to Put Them Out?*	08
2. OUR WIDGETS TALK *And They Have Some Really Valuable Things to Say*	22
3. CULTURE AND STRATEGY: A POWERFUL ALLIANCE *If You Think You've Heard This Before, Think Again*	37
4. A CHALLENGE THAT CHANGED EVERYTHING . . . FOR GOOD *The Chest Pain Project—No Budget. No Team.* *Just Eight Simple Steps.*	51
5. TURNING OUR MODEL ON ITS HEAD *People, Processes, Technology*	75
6. OUR MOST POWERFUL TOOL *You Don't Need a Manual to Use Synthetical Thinking*	87

7.	DOING IS BELIEVING *The Cycle of Transformation in Real Life*	99
8.	HEALTHCARE BEYOND RECOGNITION *Change Isn't "Transformation" Until It's Permanent*	114
9.	SAVING THOUSANDS OF LIVES & MILLIONS OF DOLLARS *This Is Transformation You Can Count*	127
10.	MOONSHOT INNOVATIONS *Rewards from Exploring the Frontier of Healthcare*	142
11.	EARTHQUAKES ARE COMING *We Can Either Brace for Them or Break New Ground Ourselves*	155
12.	HEATING HEALTHCARE FROM THE BOTTOM UP *A Handful of People Can Influence Thousands*	164
13.	THE FUTURE HOSPITAL . . . TODAY *From Doctor's Workshop to Focused Factory to Customized Care*	174
14.	THE ULTIMATE QUESTION *Are You Ready to Transform Healthcare for Good?*	180
	EPILOGUE	186

READY FOR MORE?	188
APPENDIX	190
ACKNOWLEDGMENTS	212
ABOUT THE AUTHORS	214
ABOUT THE PUBLISHER	218
ENDNOTES	222
INDEX	224
RESOURCES	232

Foreword

What if every patient received the kind of focused personal attention Dr. Kuhlman used with three US presidents? In *Transformative Healthcare*, Kuhlman and Peach show how you can provide this level of care now.

I've been on a twenty-five-year journey to make the experience of healthcare better for patients and for those who deliver care. I'm utterly convinced that patients will get the care they need only if the people delivering it get the care *they* need. Different kinds of care, equally essential. My journey began with, and has been strengthened by, being inches away from unnecessary patient deaths. Not only the ones heard about, but the ones experienced. They all happened because of a lethal brew—human fallibility as it unfolds within a complex system. The child who died after a routine colonoscopy, the cause apparently the polyethylene glycol ingested that wasn't right. The mom who had a respiratory arrest and died twenty-four hours after giving birth, the cause a combination of opioids she received and a hint of an unsavory partner. The older man who oozed to death during a thoracic aorta aneurysm repair, the cause an extended cross-clamp time and blood losing its ability to clot.

Those of us who do this work are shaped by such cases. They force us to sharpen the concepts as we do the research, make the insights more widely applicable, and most enjoyably, take action. The sketches scribbled on paper in the 1990s are now technologies that AdventHealth has actively applied across their systems. They're working. Kuhlman—navy physician, White House physician, senior flight surgeon for Marine One, hospital executive—continuously inquisitive and always skeptical, has embraced this work and made it better. Peach brings to the effort wisdom gained from his long experience running a complex multinational business. AdventHealth has been at the forefront of thinking about enterprise-wide high reliability and is reaping the reward. It hasn't been simple. It has required trust, friendship, lots of discussion, innumerable tests, some failures, and much reflection.

With Kuhlman and Peach, the discussions aren't about specific patients or cases. The conversations are dispassionate. Safe, reliable, and outstanding patient-centered care is the goal, but what we discuss while sitting together are the system characteristics and the individuals who will be needed in service of achieving safe and reliable operational excellence. We know the goals: engaged providers, reliable care. We know the means: systematically applying concepts that create high reliability.

Kuhlman and Peach have written a book that explores and describes transformational change. They sing a duet. Kuhlman addresses the foundational activity necessary to transform an organization. Peach is the architect of the building on that foundation—how the concepts of improvement are conceptualized and applied. For example, the book explores how chest pain should be effectively managed in an emergency room. Kuhlman spends time talking about the attitudes of leaders, the design of workgroups, the sources of experience, and content knowledge. Peach describes the improvement activities themselves.

The book is timely because healthcare organizations across the globe are actively considering how to achieve high reliability. The concepts are essential to an effective industry response for emergencies such as when the COVID pandemic was raging. They are also ageless, necessary for the routine management of increasingly complex environments. AdventHealth has been thinking about high reliability transformation for a while and, as a result, was better configured to confront the COVID pestilence when it arose. What Kuhlman and Peach describe in this book—the practical way to achieve effective change and the underlying concepts to support those efforts—are essential and, ultimately, every organization will need these skills to win the war on any crisis that arises. Those who don't embrace what Kuhlman and Peach describe will fail. I have seen the differences already. For example, when the COVID pandemic was at its worst, some hospitals described the devastating effect of losing nurses, leaving a smaller cohort of workers to do more. Others created an *esprit de corps* that helped them keep their employees. The differences in their attitudes and the issues they dealt with were stark.

In the early 1990s I found myself sitting on a small wave called patient safety. It turned into a tsunami that has swept through healthcare. Many organizations and individuals have joined the challenge, surfing the increasingly taller and steeper slope of that wave. Together we gained firmer footing on the surfboard, and the results are now evident: better engagement, safer patients. Kuhlman and Peach are travelers on that journey.

Join them by reading their book. You'll become surer-footed, too. Happy reading.

Allan S. Frankel, MD
CEO, Safe & Reliable Healthcare
Author, *Strategies for Building a Hospitalwide Culture of Safety*

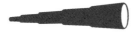

Introduction

This Is Our Purpose

From the year 2000 to 2013, Dr. Jeffrey Kuhlman engaged in the type of patient-first care that only a handful of doctors will ever experience. His patients: Presidents Bill Clinton, George W. Bush, and Barack Obama. Politics had no place in Kuhlman's work. Neither did agendas or budgets or quotas or standard processes. His duty: never be more than two minutes away from the president at any given time. Always treat him with the best care possible in his time of need.

Kuhlman needed to know the personal habits and medical histories of each president. He had to listen. He had to be focused. He had to be prepared for any situation that might arise. The experience began to rekindle Kuhlman's passion for medicine. What he did for the presidents, their families, and for senior officials is what healthcare should be like for patients who don't live in the White House or travel on Air Force One—in other words, the patients we see every day.

After coming to AdventHealth as senior vice president and associate chief medical officer, Kuhlman used an overarching question to guide his quest to transform healthcare in a meaningful way: "What if everyone in healthcare (doctors, administrators, nurses, maintenance workers, everyone) treated each patient with the kind of focus and personal attention that a physician uses with the president of the US?" We could save more lives. We could improve the overall well-being of more patients. We'd be reminded of why we wanted to get into healthcare in the first place.

Now that would truly be transformative.

It so happened that Daniel Peach had been considering a similar question after taking on his role as director of clinical transformation for AdventHealth: How can we cut through processes and excess data to reestablish a true patient-first mindset?

A registered osteopath in the United Kingdom, Peach has expertise in prevention, care, and optimizing performance of elite athletes. But his career has also included personal security for VIPs and more than twenty years as an executive for an international fiber-optic telecommunications company. In every facet of his career, Peach has seen firsthand that the most in-depth data and the greatest technology the world has ever seen are all meaningless unless they're tied to a genuine customer experience. And that is perhaps the most crucial link in transforming healthcare: relationships.

So, is it possible? Can we really transform healthcare as we know it? Kuhlman and Peach wouldn't be writing this book if all they had were another theoretical exercise. They're actually doing it. Here, they provide a method that any group can implement.

If you still think transformation is too big of a task, think of this: the drastic change outlined in this book began with three people and no budget. It has since saved thousands of lives and millions of dollars. The method is easy to follow, quick to initiate change, and powerful beyond their expectations. Doctors and administrators believe in it. So does each person who has been affected at the heart of our work: the patient. And we should all agree, that's the bottom line that matters most.

From the Authors—Transformed: Skeptics to Believers

"It sounds like an impossible task: transform healthcare. I'm here to tell you it isn't. Admittedly, I was skeptical when our boss challenged us to make significant changes to the way we deliver care and to save lives and money. But with the input of scores of physicians and nurses, my colleague Daniel Peach and I have developed specific strategies that anyone in any healthcare organization can implement. As a doctor, father, husband, and researcher, I'm now excited about the future of healthcare. We can make it more affordable, more effective, and more personal. And it only takes a few people to ignite the spark."
— **Jeffrey Kuhlman, MD, MPH**

"Here's the hard truth: Healthcare is too expensive, and too many people are dying. The good news? We can make effective change quickly and permanently by shifting our primary focus from systems and technology to what's right in front of us: relationships. They're the foundation of whole-person health. So, how can relationships save thousands of lives and millions of dollars? There's a method to it. Our teams have implemented the method. They've seen the results. It's permanently changing the effectiveness of our work, starting at the front lines. And that's why we can honestly say we're excited about the future of healthcare."
— **Daniel J. Peach**

CHAPTER 1

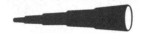

Our Beds Are on Fire

So Why Are We Waiting for Someone Else to Put Them Out?

It's a clear, dark night, 40,000 feet above the Atlantic Sea and halfway between continents. Of all the experiences I (Jeff) had as the physician to the presidents of the United States, this is one of the most memorable. We're flying on Air Force One and I've settled in for a nice trip after making sure everyone else is taken care of. There are two medical personnel aboard the plane: a critical care nurse and myself. In my role, I'm never to be more than two minutes away from the president at any given moment in case anyone has a medical event. On this particular night, we're heading to a summit of world leaders and nothing is out of the ordinary.

I'd traveled many times in motorcades and on Air Force One with three different presidents, oftentimes with their senior executive teams and occasionally with the first families of the US. You get to know each other pretty well when you travel together, and from a doctor's perspective there are few things more valuable than an established relationship with a patient—president or not.

It's an hour or so into the flight. As is usually the case at night, it's quieter than you might think for an airliner carrying people tasked with making critical national decisions day in and day out. And then a Secret Service agent taps me on my shoulder, kneels down beside my seat, and in a hushed voice says, "Hey, doc. We need you."

> Maybe the most powerful force is a mindset, a fresh way of thinking, led by the people at the bedside.

I know right away this isn't about a sniffle or a foot cramp. Over the Secret Service agent's shoulder, I can see a senior official who's obviously experiencing serious discomfort. We'd been familiar enough with the medical history of this senior official that I always had a little cautionary voice in the back of my head saying, "I hope he's never on a transatlantic flight with us at night."

Sure enough, there he is, complaining of chest pain.

If I had no knowledge of this senior official's history, the most accepted protocol at this altitude would be to put an oxygen mask over his face, tell the pilot to find the nearest airport, and land the plane. We'd take him to a hospital. The medical team there would do a series of tests. They would use every type of technology available to rule out the worst case, no matter the ramifications. In other words, they'd follow the same pattern that most doctors would follow with any patient in any hospital across the US.

This, however, is Air Force One. If we divert course and land for a possible emergency, everyone on both sides of the ocean will know about it—and at this point, for all I know, the senior official could be experiencing gas pain, acid reflux, or any number of relatively minor ailments. Rather than confer with the pilot, I first take a long look at the senior official and go through a series of questions in my mind: Does this look or sound like he's having the big one? Could it be a mild heart attack? Or might it be indigestion?

Then I take a few seconds to talk with the senior official, who is now a patient, and evaluate his symptoms and history. He's a little younger than middle age. I'm familiar with his risk factors for heart disease and with any likelihood that he might have elevated blood pressure, blood sugar, or cholesterol. I know how active he is, whether he smokes, and what he had for dinner. Prior to this trip, we'd just received a handheld test where we can poke your finger, draw a drop of blood, and check the cardiac enzyme to see if there's any indication of a heart attack. The test is clean. For good measure, there on the plane we hook him up to a 12-lead electrocardiogram. Fortunately, I know how to read the results of the EKG. It's normal, too.

After sorting everything together and engaging him in as much conversation as he feels up to, I have no reason to believe that coronary artery disease or a heart attack is causing the chest pain. I treat the senior official for alternate causes of the discomfort and monitor him into the night. We continue on the flight.

A few hours later we successfully land and no one outside Air Force One knows that someone on board had chest pain, let alone any speculation of a heart attack. We avoid an international incident—and there's no telling how costly that would have been.

The story of what happened that night on Air Force One is a continual reminder of why I went into medicine in the first place—and I'm certainly not an outlier. Most physicians can look back at the essays we wrote on our medical school applications and see common themes, perhaps in an order something like this:

- We want to heal individuals.
- We want to make people healthier.
- We want to take diagnostic challenges and offer patients leading-edge treatments whenever necessary.

It's hard to explain the joy and satisfaction of fully engaging with a person, evaluating his or her condition, and tapping into personal knowledge to determine the most effective solution . . . and watching that person walk out the door, feeling better.

The incident with the senior official on Air Force One has become a reminder for me that each of us in healthcare should treat every patient with the same type of personal attention and the same kind of relationship that I provided the official. It should be happening in emergency departments, primary-care facilities, and hospital rooms. What happened that night over the Atlantic Ocean should not be an unusual approach to healthcare. It should exemplify healthcare everywhere.

The questions I asked for several years: how do we get from where we are in healthcare today to where we need it to go? What's the force that can change the direction of this train? We've tried new systems and directives handed down from domed capitol buildings and corporate offices. Maybe the most powerful force is a mindset, a fresh way of thinking, led by the people at the bedside.

Think about it. Now *that* would be different. It would be transformative.

Health . . . Care: Have We Forgotten What It Means?

In recent decades healthcare in the US has taken a turn—and let's be honest, it hasn't been a good turn. If you were to survey twenty people in your community, how many would say they really like where we are currently with healthcare? How many would say they like where we seem to be headed?

Chest pain is a good example of one of the forks we face in the road. Earlier in my career, I worked in emergency departments at several different hospitals. Wherever I went, the ratio stayed pretty consistent: about one in ten patients who come in for emergencies are complaining of chest pain. In my early years, everyone in emergency care learned to quickly sort through hunches based on one's experience, expertise, and certain guidelines to determine if a patient was having a heart attack or might be on the verge of having one. You'd add it all up and treat them appropriately.

At some point, however, we started going in a totally different direction. Healthcare simply became an industry or a system or a business model. The change started at the top and seeped into every area of care, including chest-pain cases in emergency departments. What we described above as the most effective personal method to treat chest pain didn't align too well with a systematic approach. Neither did most of healthcare as we once knew it.

Healthcare by its very definition is not intended to be an "industry." It lives up to its name only when we all have the burning passion to make the patient our first, second, and third priorities.

We really don't have a choice. Healthcare as we know it in the US has to be transformed—permanently changed. And that means we need to break from the status quo and face head-on the problems that interfere with our top priorities—the problems we see every day in healthcare.

HEALTH CONSUMPTION EXPENDITURES PER CAPITAL U.S. DOLLARS, PPP ADJUSTED

United States	$10,966
Switzerland	$7,732
Germany	$6,646
Austria	$5,851
Sweden	$5,782
Netherlands	$5,765
Comparable Country Average	$5,697
Belgium	$5,428
Canada	$5,418
France	$5,376
Australia	$5,187
Japan	$4,823
United Kingdom	$4,653

Notes: U.S. value obtained from National Health Expenditure data. Health consumption does not include investments in structure, equipment, or research.

Source: KFF analysis of OECD and National Health Expenditure (NHE) data

Per Person Spending, Country Comparison, Peterson-KFF Health System Tracker, 2019

Our Two Hottest Fires

Let's start with the most obvious problem with healthcare in the United States: *it's way too expensive*. Americans spend an average of nearly $10,000 per person every year on healthcare[1]—for many, it's much more than that amount—and the number is continually rising. The personal costs are more than they are in any other country in the world. That should be alarming enough.

Unfortunately, we have a second critical problem, one that we should not have, given how much money Americans are paying for healthcare: *too many people in the US die too early*. The Central Intelligence Agency (CIA) ranks the United States 43rd in the world in terms of life expectancy, right among the islands of Turks and Caicos and the islands of Wallis and Futuna.[2] Needless to say, the citizens of those island nations are not paying anywhere near what Americans are paying for healthcare. Perhaps it's because they do not have to fight a gauntlet of systems and approvals simply to receive the care necessary to survive.

It is not a great scenario in a country so advanced when something as important as healthcare is 1) too costly and 2) too ineffective.

This is why we say healthcare as a whole is literally on fire. As conversations take place in boardrooms and government offices, everything from basic treatments to long-term care is becoming more and more expensive, while people are dying before they should. How can this be? We have the best technology. We have piles of data. We've even become adept at streamlining procedures and continually perfecting protocols. And yet the healthcare we're so passionate about continues to burn before our very eyes.

FIRST 50 COUNTRIES IN TERMS OF LIFE EXPECTANCY

Rank	Country	Years	Rank	Country	Years
1	Monaco	89.40	28	Cayman Islands	81.84
2	Singapore	86.19	29	Isle of Man	81.84
3	Macau	84.81	30	Bermuda	81.83
4	Japan	84.65	31	Belgium	81.65
5	San Marino	83.68	32	Slovenia	81.61
6	Canada	83.62	33	Finland	81.55
7	Iceland	83.45	34	Puerto Rico	81.47
8	Hong Kong	83.41	35	Denmark	81.45
9	Andorra	83.23	36	Ireland	81.45
10	Israel	83.15	37	Germany	81.30
11	Guernsey	83.03	38	United Kingdom	81.30
12	Switzerland	83.03	39	Portugal	81.29
13	Malta	83.00	40	Greece	81.28
14	Australia	82.89	41	Saint Pierre and Miquelon	81.20
15	Korea, South	82.78	42	Faroe Islands	81.04
16	Luxembourg	82.78	43	Taiwan	80.95
17	Italy	82.67	44	Turks and Caicos Islands	80.60
18	Sweden	82.60	45	Wallis and Futuna	80.45
19	Jersey	82.43	46	**United States**	**80.43**
20	France	82.39	47	Saint Barthelemy	80.36
21	Lichtenstein	82.36	48	Saint Martin	80.36
22	Norway	82.35	49	Saint Helena, Acension, and Tristan da Cunha	80.25
23	New Zealand	82.33			
24	Spain	82.21			
25	Austria	82.07			
26	Anguilla	82.00	50	Gibraltar	80.20
27	Netherlands	81.95			

The World Factbook 2021. Washington, DC: Central Intelligence Agency, 2021.
www.cia.gov/the-world-factbook/field/life-expectancy-at-birth/country-comparison

Fanning the flames is the troubling fact that paying for insurance premiums, medicines, deductibles, and office visits has become so expensive that people often choose not to seek medical care at all. Many live in constant fear of receiving an exorbitant bill. Health, then, has become a gamble. Care is often out of reach. This is the all-too-common scenario in many families:

"Honey, you don't look so well."

"Well, actually, I'm not feeling great."

"This has been going on for a while. It might be something serious."

"Yeah, I've thought about that."

"Let me take you to the hospital, or at least to the doctor."

"Hospital? Doctor? No, no, no. Let's wait. We can't afford that. I might be OK."

Might be OK. It's happening all around us every day. People are paying so much out of their pockets, just to carry an insurance card and maybe pay for everyday prescriptions, that they put off everything else. Ignore the symptoms. Wait and see. I can't pay for all those tests. We might expose ourselves to a system that's going to cost us our house and our life savings.

Is it any wonder that people in the US go broke because of the healthcare system?[3] Or worse, that they become seriously ill and potentially die to avoid the cost of it?[4]

Where We Are:
The Tech and Data Approach

Look around your hospital. Or just look in your pocket. Technology is everywhere. We could not have imagined twenty years ago this amount and this level of technology we now have at hand. With it comes endless streams of information or, to use a favorite medical term, "data."

In our hospitals, data has evolved to have two very different meanings:

Typically, administrators refer to data before making important business decisions, such as purchasing equipment or making capital investments. The thought is, if we have the most advanced tools and the best facilities, the better it will be for the patient—and for business. Data drives the decisions.

Then there are physicians and nurses, who associate data with the clinical procedures and outcomes in their daily work. This group uses information to build patient profiles and to standardize care in some respects. The thought is, if we can develop protocols based not so much on each individual case but on a systematic approach, the better the outcome for patients as a whole. Data drives these decisions as well.

As you can see, administrators and clinicians are using similar language, but we're talking about two different objectives. For executives, data equates to a set of administrative information (i.e. claims, length of stay, charges, etc.). For clinicians, data equates to clinical information (i.e. disease specific, risk adjusted, complications, etc.). While we all *think* we're doing what's best for the patient, the truth is that the patient is caught in the middle of a language chasm. Essentially, it's a conflict where no one wins. If anything, an overabundance of data often gets in the way of making the wisest decisions for the best care of patients. We need the right data at the right time in the right place—more is not better; data rich, information poor.

> Imagine if we knew each patient's health as well as a physician on Air Force One knows the health of the president.

This would be a great time for everyone to be on the same page. Otherwise, our beds will burn hotter and our patients will suffer even worse consequences.

Where We Need to Be: The Synthetical Approach

In the months and years following my personal healthcare experiences with the presidents, their families, and their teams, I (Jeff) attempted to harness that kind of care, expand it, and give it a name. It wasn't until Danny and I were given permission to break old paradigms that we defined our new approach as this: *synthetical thinking*.

It sounds lab-centric, but it's precisely the opposite. The synthetical approach is simple and personal. It's what physicians and nurses know is best, even as they've been restricted from using it. Obscure as the term *synthetical thinking* might be, the meaning of it has become the hot ember from which we've begun to transform the care that our teams deliver.

We'll discuss much more about synthetical thinking throughout this book, particularly in chapter six. For now, we can all agree that healthcare—or more accurately, the practice of medicine—comes down to a blend of information and relationships. So far in the 21st century we've become consumed with information. Because of that, we've lost touch with the importance of relationships. Some people will deny this. But be honest. We do a good job of *talking* about relationships, whether it's the administrator-clinician relationship or the clinician-patient relationship. But for the most part the talk is simply lip service.

The reality is we're in love with technology and data, so much so that we might not recognize how we're pushing our one-on-one relationships to the side.

The most valuable doctor-patient relationship includes observation, asking questions, and empathy—all of it helping the doctor to glean individual input for care. This relationship is at the core of synthetical thinking. We cannot look to a test (technology) or the electronic medical record (data) as the brain that directs how a patient will be treated. The person caring for that patient is the brain, the thinker. By recapturing that kind of accountability through synthetical thinking, we'll restore the care and the trust that has diminished over the years.

We would certainly start to put out some of the fires. And we'd see evidence of transformation from all perspectives—administrators, clinicians, and patients.

This Is the Perfect Time for a New Direction

There's the word again: transformation. Yes, it's overused these days. We hesitate to use it ourselves. But there's no better way to describe the opportunity in front of us. Rest assured, we aren't interested in generating yet another buzz around a vague concept. The transformation we're talking about in healthcare can be enacted right now. This change will require everyone to collaborate like a brigade to collectively put out our fires. It will necessitate like-mindedness from the front lines and the front offices to utilize information, but never in isolation. We all need to point back to genuine relationships.

Earlier in this chapter we mentioned where the US ranks in life expectancy relative to two island nations. Certain small nations and islands around the world rank even higher. When you travel to those places, you notice right away how the people who live there approach relationships. They'll say, "When Americans ask, 'How are you?' we know they don't really want a thoughtful answer. It's just a greeting so they can move on. But when people who live here ask, 'How are you?' it means we're willing to stop and take time for a conversation because we truly care how you're doing."

Strange as it sounds, maybe we can learn something from that example. Imagine if we knew each patient's health as well as a physician on Air Force One knows the health of the president and each senior official. Imagine using data and technology to *complement* individual care rather than to drive it. Imagine a return to patient-centric medicine. No doubt we could cut unnecessary costs and help people live longer and healthier.

> Are you ready—*really* ready—to lead the kinds of change we all want to see in healthcare?

This is not simply pie in the sky. The methodologies you see in the following chapters are more detailed and more proven than concepts pulled from the ether. The two of us have found *and used* a concrete methodology that anyone in healthcare can easily learn, implement, and adjust to make it their own. We have outcomes to prove this methodology lowers costs and saves lives. In fact, as we were working on this book, peer reviewers for *The Lancet* published an article about the methodologies we used to transform our care for chest pain in our hospitals. The paper included the striking results from a short sample period. We'll fully explain the findings published in *The Lancet* in chapter four (the entire article is at the back of this book), but we also want to stress that the recognition and subsequent groundswell of support in the medical field, frankly, was not our initial motivation. Our goal was simply to get back to doing what's best for the patient—somehow, some way. It just so happens, that's exactly what is needed to transform healthcare.

So ask yourself before you dive in: Are you ready—*really* ready—to lead the kinds of change we all want to see in healthcare?

If so, then brace yourselves. We're about to head in directions you didn't expect.

KEY POINTS FROM CHAPTER ONE

- **Remember our purpose.** We all entered healthcare with a passion to heal individuals and make them healthier. Keep the focus.

- **Healthcare, simplified.** Healthcare lives up to its name only when we all have the burning passion to make the patient our first, second, and third priorities. It's about the "health" and "care" of people—not an industry buzzword.

- **Two glaring challenges.** Healthcare in the United States has become too expensive, and too many people die prematurely. We need to actively engage these challenges.

- **Our focus is off target.** Technology and data are two valuable resources, but we've become too infatuated with them. The patient should be the priority over technology.

- **The solution: synthetical thinking.** This term isn't found in a textbook or a dictionary, but the source of the solution is found in synthetical thinking.

- **Our most urgent call.** Change helps extinguish the fires and saves lives and money.

REFLECTIONS

- Write down why you want to be a provider of patient care.
- Record the 2–3 barriers that are getting in your way.

CHAPTER 2

Our Widgets Talk

And They Have Some Really Valuable Things to Say

One of our favorite cartoon tropes is the classic scene of a doctor who has just entered a patient's room. The man on the examining table has an arrow through his head. There are all kinds of funny captions that have been written of how the doctor addresses the patient. We liked this setup so much that we created two versions of the cartoon ourselves. We'll share one now and one later. In our first example, our physician, with his eyes dutifully fixed on the tablet in his hand, says, "So . . . what seems to be the problem?"

Years ago, this cartoon might have seemed outlandish. But it is now emblematic of where we are in healthcare today. It's certainly the perception of the patients. But the reality of that cartoon is no less frustrating for the doctors who entered the field of medicine for the purpose of helping people live healthier, one patient at a time. The humor of the cartoon points to the core of what we need to transform: focusing our attention on the doctor-patient interaction rather than on the technology, tests, and data we have so easily accessible at hand.

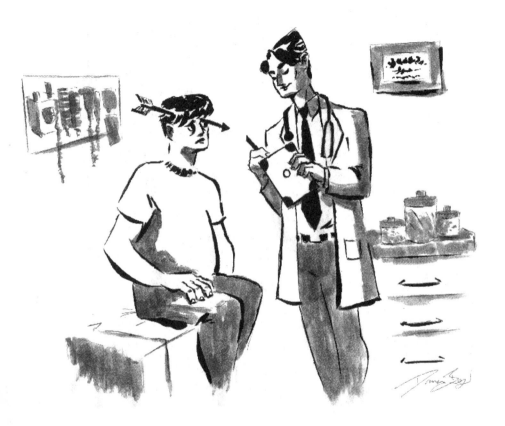

"So . . . what seems to be the problem?"

This really struck a chord with me (Jeff) when I went to a doctor's appointment with my father-in-law not long ago. He was starting to have some memory loss issues. After we filled out all the paperwork, the nurses took us back to record my father-in-law's blood pressure and vitals, and then to enter all the demographic information into their medical records system. A few minutes later, the doctor entered the patient room and sat at the desk without facing us. He looked at his computer screen and started filling out all the data fields. I knew what was happening. He was going through a checklist of what his employer required him to do and what the government also required of his employer. If he doesn't follow the checklist, then his practice stands a chance of losing some reimbursement or losing points on quality scores.

This doctor most likely wanted very much to walk into that room, look at my father-in-law, and start a conversation with both of us about his history and his health risks. He could have learned significant information about my father-in-law by asking simple questions like, "What did you have for breakfast? What are the names of your children? Are you experiencing any frustration when trying to perform basic tasks for daily living?" Even if he'd never heard the term *synthetical thinking*, that's exactly what he likely *wanted* to use to help my father-in-law. And that would have been far more helpful in making an accurate diagnosis and to formulate a specific game plan. Data could have helped in the synthetical approach, too. Instead, the data became *everything*.

The interaction, or lack of it, made me realize something profoundly true: at the end of the day, data and technology don't really care about my father-in-law. If anything, they simply get in the way.

Two Caregiver Perspectives

As a physician myself, I could sympathize with the doctor in the office that day. He knew he had precisely 8.6 minutes to fill out 72 data fields. The completion of those on-screen forms would determine his value as a medical practitioner to the healthcare system. Patient after patient, day after day, week after week... this is how a doctor is judged. The process of the inputting of data becomes directly tied to his or her self-worth. Yes, those who go into medicine have different personality types. Some thrive on the complexity of data and acquisition of technology. But unless the data and technology are used to complement firsthand evaluation, then it's just 8.6 minutes and 72 data fields, over and over.

Ask yourself: Does this sound like effective *healthcare*?

When you're on the receiving end, either personally or as a caregiver for a loved one, this issue becomes crystal clear. You suddenly see the best decisions will probably not be made unless you literally pull the doctor away from the tablet and say, "Hey, doc, *look*. He has an arrow sticking through his head. The problem is right here in front of you; the words you're typing into the system aren't helping him."

ANATOMY OF A DOCTOR'S VISIT

THE VISIT	TODAY'S HEALTHCARE	TRANSFORMED HEALTHCARE
Time in Patient Room	15 minutes	15 minutes
Primary Focus	72 data fields	1 patient
Time Observing/ Listening	6.4 minutes	15 minutes

Again, it isn't the choice of doctors to stare at those screens. The directive comes from far beyond the walls of the patient rooms. Don't get us wrong. Data and technology have allowed us to advance patient care to where it takes a patient two hours rather than a week to recover from hernia surgery. We can replace a hip and watch a patient walk within days. But some of the successes have driven us into a bubble where we surround ourselves in the aura of data and technology. They have even been the focal points of a movement called, ironically enough, "healthcare transformation."

Healthcare Transformation 1.0: A Mulligan

At some level, the desire to change the way healthcare is delivered has been constant. Make it more effective. Help people heal faster. Find ways to improve overall health. Make a positive difference on society.

The concept of "healthcare transformation" gained a lot of traction in the 1990s as insurance companies, attorneys, pharmaceutical executives, and government leaders got more involved in healthcare as an industry. Hospital administrators saw threats to traditional healthcare delivery and to established business models. And so, they looked for new answers for the new challenges. The best answers, according to some leaders, would have to come from successful work far removed from age-old norms of healthcare.

Around that time, several high-profile hospital organizations sent representatives way outside the box to learn lessons from an unlikely source: the manufacturing industry. Bells chimed and light bulbs clicked as those reps returned to their teams with ideas to implement "lean" practices into the healthcare setting.

Almost overnight, Toyota became kind of a gold standard in healthcare.[5] The company combined quality, value, and profit in a way other automakers could never quite mimic. What started with the Toyota template then extended to visits to other industrial manufacturers known to be the hallmarks of efficiency—makers of airplanes, snowmobiles, and smaller widgets. Those experiences were then shared through journals and books and conferences. We started to hear a new vernacular in our own administrative offices: Six Sigma, lean processes, standardization, the perfect experience. Any administrator who didn't embrace "lean" risked being called arrogant or old school.

> Here's the problem with using lean manufacturing concepts in healthcare: Our widgets talk. They're called patients.

The concepts came at an appropriate time. Healthcare needed something new to cross over to the 21st century. Streamlining supplies, eliminating waste, moving patients more easily—much of this has been learned from examples in manufacturing facilities. It's easy to see why these changes were so easily hailed as "revolutionary" and "transformative" in healthcare. No question, they have helped us move forward.[6]

But we've taken it too far.

Lean manufacturing is great for widget making. If you want to use the best method to turn one sheet of metal into five colanders, then you might be wise to use tools and techniques learned from Six Sigma—which is, essentially, a statistical method using data to continuously improve a product. It's a way to reduce defects and analyze results. You can scale down the materials needed to make the colander. You can shorten the time that each piece flows through production. You can invest in new robotics and machinery to punch the holes. Success is based on making the widgets at a lower cost. Ideally, the quality goes up—be it an automobile part, a windscreen on a snowmobile, or a roll of tin foil.

No matter how *lean* is presented, in healthcare we've mostly used it for increasing efficiency for the sake of profit. The true purpose of Lean Thinking, a term coined by James P. Womack and Daniel T. Jones in the early 2000s,[7] is that lean is customer focused on what would provide value to the customer (patient) via the elimination of unnecessary steps in the process of providing the value the customer seeks—hence, reduction of waste in healthcare would equate to greater margins in profit. Or so it seemed it would. Just as there are 72 data fields to fill out during a typical patient visit, in lean the indirect effect in the pursuit of efficiency in healthcare resulted in, to no one's surprise, more data and more technology taking us further away from direct patient care.

> Unlike a widget, everyone at the front line can talk. And the information they provide is priceless.

Here's the problem with using lean manufacturing concepts in healthcare: Our widgets talk. They're called patients. Every single one of them is different. So we shouldn't be treating them like widgets at all. As the following illustration shows, Human-Centered Work is at the heart of the transformation. In healthcare we worked the foundations of standardization—visuals, having supplies "Just in Time," error-proofing critical surgeries, and marching in unison toward continual improvement. However, we missed the bigger picture. We, the humans at the heart of healthcare—the physicians, nurses and frontline staff that ultimately provide direct patient care—were all so focused on becoming the next Toyota of healthcare that we developed more systems, gathered more data, and implemented more informational technologies. But we lost sight of our true customer-focused initiative toward patient care.

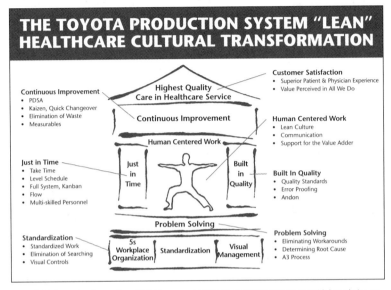

© 2009 GP Strategies Corporation. All rights reserved. GP Strategies and GP Strategies with logo design are registered trademarks of GP Strategies Corporation.[8]

Are We Listening?

When the doctor treated my (Jeff's) father-in-law for his memory-loss issues, whatever he read on the computer screen most likely provided some direction toward a diagnosis and treatment. Key word: *some* direction. If my father-in-law were a Toyota Camry, the information that was spit back out would have been enough—replace an oxygen sensor or check the air intake system. But no computer program or textbook can tell us everything we need to know about a patient. A person is not a folded piece of sheet metal. Even the best doctors with great intentions sometimes forget that fact because we're so wrapped up in the complexities of a much bigger entity.

Among the general public, healthcare is often referred to as an industry or a system rather than medical practice. This is a relatively new way of thinking, perhaps aligning with the implementation of lean manufacturing processes. We enter data into all those fields to build a process that's best for the system and, supposedly, best for all patients as a whole. But unlike a widget, this patient is not the same as *that* patient—even if they look alike and have similar symptoms.

In other words, we need to be caring for each patient with synthetical thinking—where the caregiver absorbs subjective and objective feedback from all types of sources, and then creates a tailor-made game plan for that patient.

The problem we now see is in the application of lean in healthcare; the system comes with too narrow of a focus. Business leaders are enamored with improving efficiencies and profit, and there's nothing wrong with that. We should be as efficient as possible. We need finances and resources to do the best work possible. Lean is by no means perfect but requires cultural change, which most organizations do not address, thus they lack successful understanding, deployment, and sustainment. Too often lean has been poorly deployed. Lean starts with a cultural transformation—not solely tools for efficiency. Most US companies fail at lean with low long-term adoption. People focus on tools and not on culture first. Allowing frontline staff to be engaged and empowered daily to come up with solutions is the foundation of sustainment in a lean program.

A hospital team cannot continually implement lean standards or rely on Six Sigma formulas to judge its own success. We are judged one patient at a time and as an aggregate of those patients.

The books on transforming, or reforming, healthcare talk about putting the patient first. They even claim we're listening ... but exactly who, or what, are we listening to? If we're truly going to make meaningful change, then we need to be tuned into what's going on with each patient. We need to be empathetic about the cost of proper care. We should be aware of the fact that people should be living longer, healthier lives. The patient-physician relationship—not data and how we process it—will be the number-one catalyst in the type of transformation where everyone wins.

The Most Priceless Information Is in Front of You

Let's say we all agree on the obvious: the patient is the key to transforming healthcare. With that, the good news is this: the solution to the problem is right in front of us. There's no need to spend months studying other industries or to spend millions of dollars developing new data-processing technology. We shouldn't even feel compelled to hire consultants to study our work and then tell us about it.

It's funny because whenever we so much as mention the idea of changing a culture, everyone takes three steps back and pretends they didn't hear anything. The task is too time-consuming, too daunting for us. And so, what do we do? We hire outside firms to do it for us.

Consultants do bring a degree of value in most situations. They provide fresh perspectives and can share lessons learned from their work in similar organizations with similar challenges. Plus, as a colleague once said, "Consultants always give us someone else to blame if things don't work out."

But the fact is, it's difficult for someone from the outside to come in and change the culture of an organization. Hiring a consulting firm to tell us how to treat our patients works a bit like this:

You walk up to a man and ask, "Excuse me, can you tell me what time it is?"

The man looks at you and says, "That's a nice watch you're wearing. Can I borrow it?"

You give him the watch, he fastens it to his wrist, and says, "I'm sorry, what was the question again?"

"I asked if you could tell me what time it is," you say.

The man looks at your watch, which is now on *his* wrist, and says, "Sure. But first you'll need to pay me twenty dollars." You hand him the money because you need to know the time. He says, "It's two o'clock. And do you know what I can do for you? If you pay me a thousand dollars, I'll let you have this nice watch."

And he sells you your own watch back.

This isn't meant to question the character of consultants. But it does illustrate how quick we are to ask others to find answers that are often at our own fingertips. When it comes to the type of transformative change we're talking about, building a budget for consultations simply isn't necessary. We don't need more data, more technology, or more consultation. Our clinicians give us all the expertise we need. And our patients give us all the information we need.

If we believe the best way to put out the fires in healthcare is to gather more information and bundle it together, then we'll be successful at exactly that: gathering more information and bundling it together. But what does having all that information accomplish? Our clinical staffs are already in pursuit of seemingly impossible metrics. They're so bogged down in numbers that the fires around us just burn hotter and go unnoticed.

The answer is much simpler. Synthetical thinking or synthetical care goes back to what doctors have known for centuries. All we really need to do is listen to the people who are in our presence. It also means listening to ourselves. Use data not so much as a one-size-fits-all guide for all patients, but in context with treating one patient and then the next one and the next one.

With that mindset, we can drastically change, or transform, healthcare by adopting two practices:

- Empower the front lines
- Hold them accountable with reasonable measures

We've seen tangible results from doing this. Instead of looking to industrial-type data or outside sources for real answers, we decided to engage our frontline physicians, nurses, emergency department clinicians, work-center personnel, and even patients. We simply ask on a regular basis, "What's the best way to do this?" Unlike a widget, everyone at the front line can talk. And the information they provide is priceless.

Culture Change Isn't as Hard as You Think

The first thing you learn on the first day of medical school is to *look*, to *listen*, and to *feel* when you examine a patient. Think about the cartoon with the guy sitting there, fully conscious, with the arrow sticking through his head. If the doctor had just looked at the patient, he would have said, "Oh, wow, you have an arrow in your head." Or if he would have listened to the patient, he would have heard the man say, "Hey, I have an arrow in my head because . . ." Even if the doctor had blindly felt around, he probably would have figured out what was wrong with this guy.

Our training in medicine told us there's an indefinite amount to learn when we observe patients and communicate with them. The interaction provides our most important data points. It's what we became passionate about when we chose healthcare for a career, because it leads to the type of whole-person healing that doesn't necessarily land in our hands via computer or consultant.

What we propose is the beginning of a dramatic shift in balance—the seeds of *real* transformation. With this, the emphasis of care relies heavily on relationships, values, and behaviors. Data and technology are used in context with each case, and never in isolation.

In short, we're talking about a recalibration of culture.

Uh-oh. There's that word. *Culture*. Before assuming this is the start of a three-year process and before calling the consultants back, hold on. We have the game plan, and we've implemented the plan ourselves. It isn't nearly as daunting as you might think. Our transformative ideas tap into what you already know and what you once were excited about. Wherever we've taken this, there's been no debate or pushback because it's what we all want. The change in culture happens organically, and oftentimes, even enthusiastically.

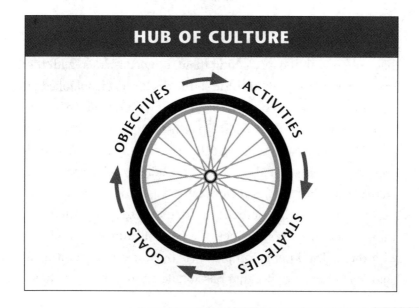

Culture is the axis on which meaningful transformation occurs. Once the culture is aligned, then your strategies, your goals, your objectives, and your activities dovetail nicely in a synergistic way. Maybe you think you've heard this before. No, you haven't. Perhaps you're skeptical about anyone who promises to dramatically change the culture and sustain it. It's OK to be skeptical. So were we.

And then we found a way to do it—quickly, affordably, and effectively. All of it with the patient in mind. We have stories and results to prove it.

KEY POINTS FROM CHAPTER TWO

- **The doctor-patient relationship.** The relationship between the physician and the patient must be at the heart of effective healthcare.

- **Those critical 15 minutes.** The patient exam needs to be a meaningful interaction between the doctor and patient rather than 15 minutes of data gathering.

- **The danger of process focus.** We work with *people*—not widgets. Excessive focus on process improvement can cause us to lose sight of our most important focus: the patient.

- **Efficient vs. effective.** Manufacturing lessons can streamline processes, but do they truly make healthcare better? The balance is imperative.

- **The obvious answer.** The best way to improve care is to pay more attention to the patient. The patient-physician relationship—not data and how we process it—will be the number-one catalyst in the type of transformation where everyone wins.

- **No outside consulting necessary.** The answer in most cases is not to bring in expensive outside consultants. Doctors, nurses, and patients know better than anyone how to make care better.

- **Culture change.** It isn't as ominous, or as expensive, as you might think. The change in culture happens organically and oftentimes enthusiastically. Change can become natural.

REFLECTIONS

- Starting tomorrow, what 2–3 changes can you implement to make your interactions with patients more meaningful?

CHAPTER 3

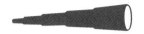

Culture and Strategy: A Powerful Alliance

If You Think You've Heard This Before, Think Again

When my son was a little younger, I (Jeff) wanted him to take out the garbage regularly. I figured it would provide a little relief for my wife and me if he'd learn to take on the job without being asked. We'd save ourselves some time. He'd become responsible. So, I did what most parents would do. I made a deal with my son: "I'll give you a dollar every time you take out the garbage."

It's the textbook approach, isn't it? Capture his attention with a little incentive and, before you know it, he'll see the value of helping around the house and of being a responsible family member. At some point he might even decide to expand on our deal.

Sure enough, it worked—or I should say, we had a positive start. Several times a week I'd see him pulling the garbage from our kitchen and hauling it outside. He didn't complain about the job, and he didn't even negotiate for more than one dollar.

As a parent, I was pretty proud of my plan and thought, "Wow, that wasn't so hard. Maybe we're ready for the next steps."

Over time, though, I realized something was missing. My son hadn't learned the bigger lesson of helping for the greater good of our family, nor would he willingly accept more responsibility for "job satisfaction." I'm pretty sure such concepts never crossed his mind. If I'd stopped paying him, he would have assumed he could stop taking out the trash. In fact, whenever we'd ask him to wash the dishes or help in the yard, he'd ask, "How much are you paying me?" For him, taking out the garbage had become a short-term means to an immediate result: a buck.

The positive results of our arrangement—a task completed; a dollar earned—applied only to one specific act for one specific reward. You could say we were caught up in the vortex of rapid-cycle improvement. In rapid-cycle improvement, you identify a problem and you find a way to solve it through routine. Often, there's a benefit.

Rapid-cycle improvement is in the same family as performance-improvement, or PI, strategies. There's little argument these types of strategies bear results. We've all been part of PI projects, professionally and personally, even if we didn't realize it at the time. Sales goals. Quotas. Salary incentives. Rewards for losing weight or for earning a good grade on a test. A short-term strategy leads to a short-term result. Repeat: *short*-term. Typically, any advantages you reap will probably fall by the wayside in a matter of weeks, months, or perhaps years. Results are finite in scope and in longevity.

That's what happened with our take-out-the-garbage strategy. We saw a performance improvement. But from a bigger-picture perspective, we never should have assumed we'd see sustained and expanded results.

PERFORMANCE IMPROVEMENT STRATEGIES	MORE OPTIMAL MANAGEMENT STRATEGIES
Identify a Short-Term Goal	Identify a Long-Term Goal
Motivate an Action to Achieve the Goal	Motivate Change in Values/Behaviors
Look at Short-Term Achievement as a Win	Continually Evaluate Sustained Change

Healthcare Is Not an Industry

Widget making gives us a vivid picture of rapid-cycle improvements. It's probably why leaders in business and healthcare have become so enamored with it. Developing a leaner manufacturing process is not that difficult, and the results will show up quickly. You can store the sheets of metal closer to the production line. You can increase the speed of cutting the sheets by 10 percent. You can make the packaging smaller. These kinds of rapid-cycle improvement are all beneficial to the business. But they don't correspond to meaningful change beyond the data on spreadsheets.

Therefore, we cannot improve healthcare, let alone transform it, by investing ourselves in the systems that work in an industrial environment. There, it's a colander or a can or a car door. It goes into a crate and is shipped off forever.

That's manufacturing. We are healthcare. A hospital is about as similar to a manufacturing facility as a human being is similar to a steering wheel.

Real transformation starts with the way we care for patients.

This is not to say that rapid-cycle improvements have no place in healthcare. We use PI all the time. We change an antibiotic to counter an infection. We reorganize supply closets to improve accessibility. Yes, the patient experience improves . . . for a while . . . and then we have to revisit those changes again.

Clinical transformations that will dramatically reduce costs and save lives need to be more than a series of lean improvements. They need to reach across a multitude of disciplines. They have to engage entire teams, keep them engaged, and be easily understood when new people join those teams. Ultimately, transformative change means cultural change, and it should be demonstrated every time we come in contact with a patient.

A prime example of this is how we've transformed our treatment of sepsis.

The Sepsis Trial

Sepsis is an overwhelming infection of the body. It happens in response to a variety of illnesses, like respiratory pneumonia or exotic blood-borne viruses like Ebola. Unstopped, sepsis can cause a patient to go into shock. The infection threatens to cascade into the vascular system, which will then lead to a struggle to sustain life. Sepsis by far is the number-one cause of in-hospital deaths in the US and globally.[9]

Traditionally, whenever we discover a patient has sepsis, we throw everything plus the kitchen sink at the infection in hopes of stopping it from worsening. Most of what we use is based off the metrics we're given—data compiled over a number of years and from hospitals across the country. Even the government weighs in by telling us to work within certain parameters. We have to pay attention to time limits and protocols, gleaned from many different performance-improvement strategies. Changing an antibiotic, however, is simply a response that will rarely save a life, as the change is usually too little, too late. Sepsis patients die due to a system-wide vascular collapse rather than as a result of an untreated infection. There is no magical next-day solution for sepsis. Basically, anytime we *react* to sepsis, we're three steps behind where we should be because reactionary care is costlier and more dangerous for the patient.

Therefore, we decided proactively to make a cultural transformation in the way we discover sepsis and treat it. Ideally, we'd reap short-term results but also allow enough input and deviations to sustain those results for the long term.

We know that treating a patient with sepsis necessitates a variety of expertise from a whole team of people, all working in sync. Think about it. Sepsis has a higher in-hospital mortality rate than heart attacks or strokes. Yet we move mountains and fly helicopters to treat heart attacks and strokes at the onset, as we should.

> Everyone on the team needs to be empowered to take action when they see the warning signs.

However, we need to do the same for sepsis. Recognition and treatment should start long before we reach the critical stage.

Let's backtrack the timeline of a patient who comes into the emergency department with a bad infection. Our initial contact might be the moment the patient is picked up on the street or at home. That should be the start of the recognition and treatment stage. So let's empower the paramedics and the EMTs to determine those first warning signs and start the proper fluids. Empower them to observe the patient and to use equipment and treatments that specifically target the patient right there in front of them. Do not shackle them to a long checklist of to-dos before they can consider the potential for sepsis. Time is too critical. The longer we wait, the more expensive the treatment options become and the less likelihood for full recovery.

So, in our plan, by the time the patient enters the emergency department, treatment for possible sepsis has started. By doing that, the attention of the doctor in the ED will *not* have to be on a computer, where he or she has to spend valuable time sifting through data and defaulting to a preset power plan. Every minute takes us closer to a tipping point.

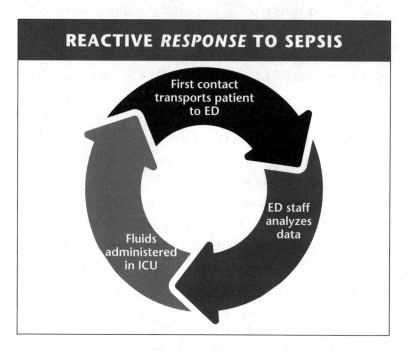

To the best of our knowledge, no lives have been saved by *ordering* an antibiotic. The medicine has to be dripping into the veins and circulating through the body, killing the organisms that are causing the overwhelming infection. Fluid resuscitation is just as important as the antibiotics at this point. The whole process needs to be happening in real time—not after all the entries have been completed on a checklist.

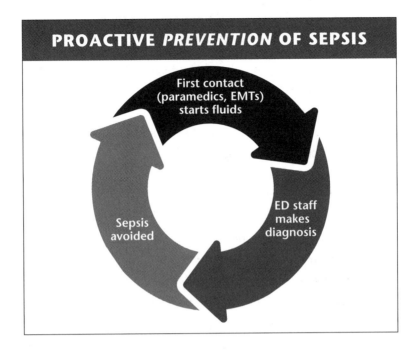

But . . . Can We Do That? Yes, We Can.

You can guess the initial response to our change in sepsis treatment. Many doctors were afraid—literally afraid—to break from the protocol that had been handed down. We remember some saying, "Whoa, we're going to put patients into heart failure." Or, "What if they go into kidney failure? Can their bodies handle the overload of fluids?"

Our answer is, "Well, they're going to die if you don't fluid resuscitate them to keep their organs performing. And if you top off the fluids a little too much, it's OK, we certainly know how to treat that."

Sepsis is one of our beds on fire. How do you respond when you smell smoke? You can leave the room and look up a presupposed set of procedures, hoping the fire doesn't burn everything down before the fire chief arrives. Or you can allow the first people who smell the smoke to pull the fire alarm and make every effort to put the fire out. It doesn't require a fire chief to inform everyone there's a fire in the bed, and neither should we wait to treat sepsis until the patient is under a physician's care in an ICU.

Everyone on the team needs to be empowered to take action when they see the warning signs. Look, listen, feel. Because information from afar doesn't tell you what an observation of the patient at your fingertips tells you: this person is on the verge of sepsis. He or she needs antibiotics and fluids.

If you don't believe the anecdotal evidence, then let's turn to the data. After we integrated this methodology in our pilot hospitals, the sepsis mortality rate dropped from 22 percent (which is around the national average) to 8 percent. The difference equates to 1,500 lives saved in two years. It's truly a win for everyone—the patients, the patients' families, and the entire healthcare team. The team sees the results. They're active participants. We're no longer assigning one task to one person. It has become our definition of a team victory: *1,500 lives*. This is not only a team victory; it really is a transformational victory.

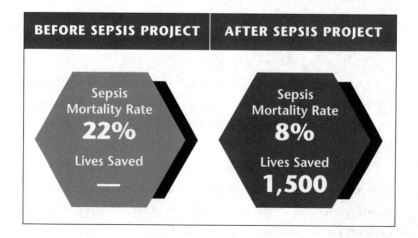

The Best Game Plan

If you watch highlights of Super Bowl LI between the New England Patriots and Atlanta Falcons, you'll see the Patriots down deep in the weeds in the second half. They trailed 28–3, and the wheels appeared to have completely fallen off.

Had the New England coaches stubbornly stuck to a game plan formulated over the previous two weeks, the contest would probably have gotten worse for the Patriots. Instead, they gathered information they'd accumulated over the course of the game, and they asked quarterback Tom Brady and the offensive linemen what they observed on the field. With that, the Patriots altered their game plan. In those now-classic highlights, the TV cameras caught Brady talking to his offensive teammates on the bench. He didn't make a passionate speech to evoke legendary stories of Vince Lombardi. He just said to every player, "Do your job. Do your job." And so, armed with an adjusted plan, each player did his job, one play at a time. The Patriots went on to make the most remarkable comeback in Super Bowl history, winning 34–28.

The same message has to be resonating if we're going to transform healthcare into what we want it to be. It's everybody doing his or her job. It's listening to the front line and especially the patient. It's empowering every person doing the work to help formulate an ever-changing plan—and holding them accountable to the plan with reasonable measures.

This is the opposite of rapid-cycle improvements where, as the name implies, quick fixes have to be made over and over and over, with a long, complex formula leading the way. There is no big idea really. Nothing big changes because the process is carved in stone. But with transformation we see dramatic change. Because when small successes snowball into huge victories, you begin to see a cultural shift from the granular level out to a grand picture.

The Coronary Artery Bypass Graft (CABG) Trial

An open-heart procedure is another high-risk area of in-patient care. Lives are either saved or lost. You're exposing the most important organ in the body, you're working around critical blood vessels, and you have the sensitivity of anesthesia; a lot is going on. A cardiothoracic surgeon must train for 10 years on coronary artery bypass grafts (CABG) before he or she can go off on their own. Given the risk of the surgery, that's probably a prudent track.

At our hospital we have ten cardiothoracic surgeons. They all do at least two isolated CABGs per week. So we have quite a bit of experience with the procedure. We can tell you the surgery takes about five hours, and we've determined a variation of the intraoperative time down to a matter of single-digit minutes.

Other healthcare systems have focused on lean or Six Sigma on the intraoperative variances. But we've found the widest and most important swing in variances from patient to patient is in the *pre*-operative and *post*-operative stages. That's where we know we can make the most difference in life-or-death decisions.

For this trial, we engaged surgeons, nurses, and recent patients to discuss what worked, what might work, and what didn't work. Without much debate we decided that the data in our system was not the most effective source to develop a holistic plan from pre-op to recovery. The computer should not make such critical decisions about the patient's well-being. Instead, the surgeons, nurses, and patients would drive the plans. And each plan would be tailored on a personalized, case-by-case basis, giving the patient his or her best possible chance of coming out of this complex operation in a better condition than they were before surgery.

That's right. We actually encouraged the medical team that would eventually be at the bedside to take the time to sit down beforehand and talk about what should be done before, during, and after the CABG surgery. They would then be tasked to follow through with the plan *and* they would be held accountable for the results—good or not so good. Those results would help them formulate a game plan for the next patient . . . and so on.

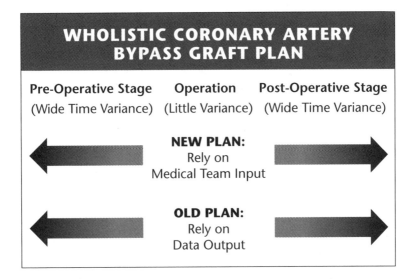

In the days before each operation, the team instructed the patient on important details that differed from person to person—and that you rarely, if ever, find in a database. When to stop using blood thinners. What type of nutrition you need (including how much to consume and when to consume it).

In addition, we shifted the paradigm at the post-op stage, which we initiate before the surgery even starts. For years, anesthesiologists would use opioids or other medications to knock patients out during surgery, and well after. But in our wholistic plan we want patients awake and back on their feet as soon as possible. The mental picture is a guy who stops mowing his lawn halfway through the job, comes in for CABG, and goes back to finish the lawn. The quicker the grass is cut, the healthier the patient.

So in this CABG pilot, our anesthesiologists determined how to give the precise amount of medication without overdoing it. We don't want to tell groggy patients, "Oh, just take it easy for a few days . . . or a week . . . or however long it takes." The last thing a heart patient needs is to be sedentary. If you rest, you rust. In the hours after surgery, instead of simply lying there, the patient would dangle their feet off the bed. Maybe they would stand with assistance. They would get their tubes and wires pulled at the appropriate time. They would drink a smoothie or whatever nutrition their stomach could tolerate to get their digestive system working again and to regain strength.

In other words, we placed our value on getting this person back to their life rather than throwing everything at the five-hour surgery itself. Everyone had a role and an objective for each particular patient—from prep all the way to the physical therapists and nutritionists.

And that's how our strategies were woven into a new culture. As we said, this defies everything we've ever heard about changing culture:

"It's costly."

"It's time-consuming."

"It might or might not take hold."

"It can't co-exist with a new strategic plan—either culture or strategy will die."

"We need more data, more data, more data."

We once had the same mindset, figuring the data-centric system was in place to protect patients and to progress them through difficult times. But now we look back and see it's slower, costlier, and much riskier.

What's interesting is that, when we sit down to talk with the medical teams about changing our approach, they all say, "This is what we've always wanted to do." They're enthused. When we discuss the plans with patients, they're happy to know our intent is for them to reach their goals—even the lofty goals. Being an active parent. Playing sports. Going back to work sooner than later. Mowing the grass. They're hopeful.

> Our story of transforming healthcare started ... with three rather nondescript people in a modest office and no budget.

The bottom line is that we're all aligned and moving toward a focused goal, with the patient taking a lead role. Patients are healthier. The process is less expensive. Beds are freed up for other critical patients who need them. We're immersed in real healthcare. For all of those reasons, it is transformative.

When we got together to discuss the framework for this book, we sat back in amazement. This chapter, for example, brings together a singular story where collaborative strategies, cultural change, and lives being saved are woven together. It's as unusual as it is powerful. Our story never once describes a quarterly executive summit. There are no teams of consultants, piles of books, or reams of data.

Our story of transforming healthcare started before the sepsis and CABG trials, with three rather nondescript people in a modest office and no budget. These people had two pillars to lean on: a creative idea and a simple eight-step process drummed up from the past.

KEY POINTS FROM CHAPTER THREE

- **Rapid-cycle improvements.** Performance-based results are easy to quantify and promote, but they've backfired in healthcare. Cultural change takes time and people.

- **The never-ending goal.** We need to look beyond immediate results and transform care for everyone's long-term good. Change is the start, not the end.

- **The sepsis trial.** We adjusted care at point of contact to save 1,500 lives. Physicians need to be empowered to question and break existing mindsets to achieve healthcare transformation.

- **The coronary artery bypass surgery trial.** We saved lives by tailoring each CABG from pre-operative stage to post-operative stage. Rely on your medical team's input to develop methodologies to address your healthcare issues.

- **Minimal resources, dramatic results.** It doesn't have to be expensive; it doesn't require teams of consultants or extensive resources.

REFLECTIONS

- Identify at least one area of patient care where the current approach is suboptimal, slow, and directs patients down an unstoppable wrong path. Make the change.

CHAPTER 4

A Challenge That Changed Everything . . . *for Good*

The Chest Pain Project—No Budget.
No Team. Just Eight Simple Steps.

We remember well the day the gauntlet came down. The chief medical officer in our hospital, Dr. David Moorhead, brought three of us together and very politely yet seriously said, "We need change. The status quo of how we've been doing things is no longer an option."

He referred to the frustrations all of us had been feeling. He hoped they would become the underpinnings of real transformation—a seismic shift—in how we treat patients. Save more lives. Make healthcare less expensive.

Of course, we thought Dr. Moorhead would back up his charge with a generous budget, a schedule of visits from consultants, and an internal executive team to offer guidance. We discovered none of the above would be coming. Instead, the three of us were sort of like the rebels in the corner, the people you didn't necessarily want to mix with because "they're the ones who want to change things." But we did have something no budget can guarantee: the blessing of our CMO to try new ideas.

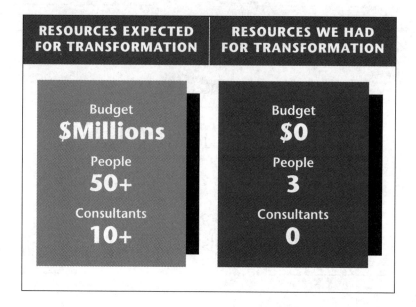

We had no certainty that our ideas, whatever they might be, would go anywhere. We privately wondered if this would simply be another exercise in futility. Two facts, however, made this challenge different: 1) we were personally and professionally invested in change, and 2) we had company in believing our mission at hand. Lots of company, it turned out.

Evidence on Our Side

Around the same time we were starting on our project, a convergence of evidence began circulating from the perceived mecca of all healthcare academics—Harvard. One particular study created quite a stir. We thought it to be quite ingenious.

In the study, researchers followed dozens of attending physicians in a hospital system considered a hallmark of "evidence-based medicine." To administrators, evidence-based medicine means if you follow guidelines rigidly without deviating, then good things will happen. When clinicians talk about evidence-based medicine, we're talking about a specific clinical approach to the practice of medicine, which might involve randomized clinical trials and evidence derived from studies.

This Harvard study showed, perhaps not surprisingly, that each physician made hundreds of decisions over the course of a workday. The surprise: fewer than 20 percent of those decisions were based on data or clinical-based evidence.[10] Remember, this is a group of hospitals we all know and respect. It's the place where patients go for the best care. Yet despite all the talk of delivering evidence-based medicine, only one in five decisions fell into that category.

> Permanent change requires patience.

So... how were the other 80 percent of the decisions made? The study found they were based on practice, experience, anecdotes, personal expertise, and remembering the warning signs from patients in the past. We call it "practice-based evidence."

The Harvard study left no doubt: practice-based evidence dominates good decision making. The report added to the concerns we had about using an overload of data and expecting physicians to stick to data and documented evidence.

Unfortunately, no one really wanted to talk about the results of the study, so it was essentially buried.

Coincidentally, a British medical journal later published an article on the same subject and came up with the same findings: only 20 percent of healthcare decisions at highly regarded UK institutions are based on evidence, and the other 80 percent are based on practice.[11] Two of the best healthcare teams on opposite sides of the ocean were seeing eye to eye on delivering the ideal care to patients. The data went completely against the trend of the past thirty years.

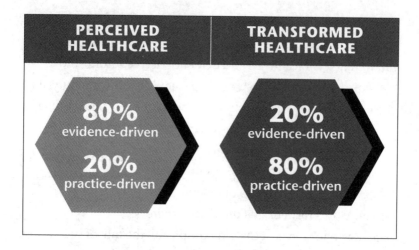

The studies galvanized what we knew in our little huddle. The healthcare system of the early 21st century, with all its metrics and data, had turned healthcare upside down. The best doctors made their best decisions based on practice and experience. The challenge for us, then, became this: How could we capture that? Could we develop a methodology where people on the front line combined experience and evidence into a structured plan that they could either 1) follow or 2) deviate from, given appropriate rationale?

If we could do that, the results might be so big and so important, no one could ignore them.

Turning Point: The Chest Pain Project

There we were, the three of us, trying to develop ideas to save lives and make healthcare less expensive. *Transform healthcare.* It's kind of lofty. We were smart enough to realize we needed help. So we gathered feedback and fanned our challenge out to colleagues. And we began to believe the emergency department might be an epicenter for a pilot project—and change.

Our hospitals see phenomenal numbers of patients in the ED. Chest pain is the number-one reason they come in—more than 100 every day, system-wide. You walk a tightrope with chest pain. The situation can be really bad . . . or it can be absolutely nothing. It can be treated with expensive tests and procedures . . . or a pill. You can admit a patient . . . or send them home. Chest pain and unanticipated admission is a huge challenge, medically *and* legally. The potential consequences persuade us to err on the side of treating for the worst possibility. Far more times than not, however, the situation isn't life or death at all. It's simply really expensive.

> Our goal isn't to be right. It's to do what's right for the patient.

And that would be our focus. How to safely and assuredly filter those patients whose lives were at stake from those who were experiencing something unrelated to a heart event. Those who needed treatment would receive full attention and resources—saving lives. Those who didn't need treatment would avoid excessive tests and evaluation—saving money.

Our first chest-pain pilots involved 400 patients. From the start we emphasized the need for some sort of methodology. But rather than turning to journals and data for a methodology, we turned to the most logical source: the front line. This would not be a rapid-cycle improvements project, where we would tell the doctors what to do and justify the process with short-term results. No, instead we invited the medical team to *lead* the change. That way, we'd gain valuable input, we'd have immediate buy-in, and the results would be long lasting.

Empowering the front line to drive the project would have a much bigger impact: it would change the culture, and the power of this changed culture would drive the process, indefinitely.

It all sounded nice. Honestly, we weren't sure it would work, let alone be accepted. We said, "The potential is too great. Let's try."

All we really had were notes about chest pain in the ED: A heart event or not a heart event. Test or don't test. Admit or release. Save patients' lives and save them money. Good for patients. Good for physicians. Good for hospitals. The notes pointed to a looming question: "How do we take these ideas from concept to reality?"

The Triad

Coalescing thoughts often revolve around thinking in threes, and our experience was no different. Our triad of thought was brought together by the need to focus on evidence and consensus-based medicine, to substantiate the clinical outcomes with data, and to incorporate that information into an innovative approach that propagated change. The triad of improvement formed the parameters around the method of change, which seated at the triad's very core, and hence became the driving force within.

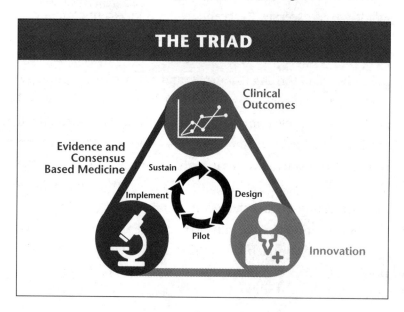

As the triad of improvement, it is important that the foundation of any cultural change should be carefully initiated around a solid basis. The triad allows the evolution of thought and evidence to collide into a structured approach built around a cyclical method, which generates the continual change and learnings of three interdependent aspects. Initially focusing on the current evidence allows for discussion and the building of a consensus of focus and adds strength to the ultimate cause. Supporting this evidence with the second cathetus allows a measure of the development of the change from a structured baseline. Finally, the innovation brings together the evidence, the data, and the true intent from a different view, based upon the want and need of the challenge. The core driver? The action—the associated driving force within from the method—that inculcates the ultimate, sustainable change from a phased systematic approach.

There are hundreds of books and lectures on Change Management 101. Many of them don't apply well to healthcare. We agreed that one, however, would: John Kotter's 8-step process for leading change. He wrote a book by that name in the 1980s and it's still considered the most complete template for changing workplaces from the inside out.

> **KOTTER'S PRINCIPLES HAVE WITHSTOOD THE TEST OF TIME BECAUSE YOU DON'T NEED AN MBA TO UNDERSTAND THE EIGHT STEPS:**

1. Establish a sense of urgency.
2. Create a guiding coalition.
3. Develop a vision and a strategy.
4. Communicate the change vision.
5. Empower employees for broad-based action.
6. Generate short-term wins.
7. Consolidate gains and produce more change.
8. Anchor your new approaches into the culture.

The book *Leading Change*, and the eight-step process, hit the bookshelves long before Amazon came along and generally around the time we saw a crisis ahead for healthcare. Executives and administrators were latching onto any reliable source for insight on how to prepare and perhaps stave off the fires.

Kotter's eight steps do not fit the processes traditionally accepted in healthcare—i.e., data-driven fixes, PI projects, quick results. So with intentionality we said, "Let's stick to these eight steps and not feel pressured to take shortcuts. However, because healthcare people might be reluctant to adopt and remember eight steps, we'll simplify them into four phases, without eliminating any of the eight steps." The four phases we developed are:

Phase 1: Design. This entails the first five steps of change management.

Phase 2: Pilot. We generate short-term wins to strengthen momentum for the final two phases.

Phase 3: Implement. Everyone helps put the plan into place and is invested in its successes.

Phase 4: Sustain. This is where groups and organizations most often fail.

For some, these phases are easier to remember and follow. But you can't jump ahead and expect meaningful results. We had one administrator ask, "Why do you spend so much time on the design?" We said, "Well, when you build a house, do you use a blueprint? Do you use designs inside and out?"

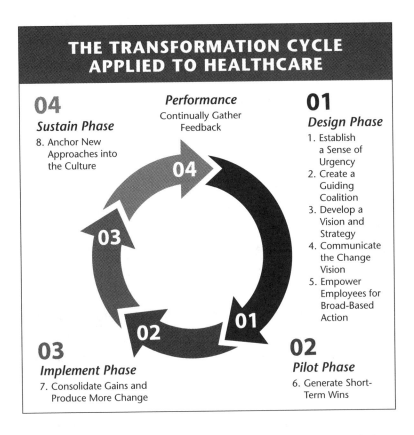

It doesn't go well if you don't have a blueprint and follow the plans, with exceptions here and there. You can throw a structure up, but it may not make it through the hurricane.

Another comment is, "Why don't you just jump to the implement phase? You know what to do." Sure, if you want a short-term victory, that might be the most expeditious thing to do. Just skip the first five steps and jump to the step where you'll see results. But be aware: it won't work for the long term. And for a need so big as transforming healthcare, we *must* reign in the temptation to see immediate successes on a quarterly report.

Permanent change requires patience. We discovered that in ways we never could have anticipated.

Step One:
A Sense of Urgency

As a general during World War II, Dwight Eisenhower famously said, "Planning is everything; the plan is nothing." We found out exactly what he meant during our chest-pain project.

The planning starts with the sense of urgency. We have 4,000 patients a month who present with chest pain in the ED (almost 50,000 patients a year). Of the 4,000, fewer than 1 percent are having an acute heart attack. We do a fantastic job of identifying those with an ST-segment elevation myocardial infarction, or STEMI. We'll whisk those straight to the cath lab within an hour where we can open up that coronary artery that's shutting down. This process is lifesaving.

For that 1 percent of patients, we'll keep doing what we're doing.

Now, what do we do with the other 99 percent who are not having a STEMI, who are not at risk of a life-threatening shutdown of the artery? Ideally, we'd sort them into those with high likelihood of having a heart attack in the next month or two, and those with no chance of having a heart attack in the next month or two.

When we started this pilot, a quarter of the patients we evaluated in the ED were deemed stable enough for discharge from the hospital. We were placing half the patients into observation status. The other quarter of the patients we admitted to the hospital. According to national norms, we were pretty conservative in keeping 75 percent of patients either for observation or admission (nationally, we found that statistic to be about 50 percent).

Those facts alone helped us establish our sense of urgency—not based on judgments or emotion but on the local information. Data helps in this first step because it reinforces to the team why we need to take this change seriously and not put it off for later.

Urgency motivates everyone to start the ball rolling. Our beds are on fire, remember?

Step Two:
Establishing Our Guiding Coalition

Let's be clear: we need smart doctors and wise executives to keep our hospitals running well. Without them, we're back to house calls. However, those are not the people who should be leading the type of change we're talking about. You need the frontline physicians for this—the emergency medicine physician, the cardiologist, the hospital medicine specialist, the doctor who works in observation units. You get them together with nursing staff because they're so deeply involved with the patients. And that's the core of your guiding coalition—the people who have their hands directly in healthcare *and* who influence others.

Keep in mind, you don't want every physician to be leading the change, because then you'd have dozens or hundreds of people and never reach any kind of consensus. You also don't need the chair of the department or the most tenured clinicians. This is not the project for academicians or researchers. You want passionate people who are excited to contribute and lead change. They're good about listening to colleagues, *and* colleagues willingly listen to them.

The first time we had eight physicians in the same room, they weren't eight physicians of the same specialty. We had two for each. They were the physicians with clinical gravitas and an ability to share their opinions in a constructive way. They had enough humility to respect everyone else on the coalition, all sharing a mindset:

Our goal isn't to be right. It's to do what's right for the patient.

Step Three:
Develop the Vision and Strategy

Once these doctors and nurses know your focal point is patient care—what's best for the patient will be best for the hospital, in that order—they're all in. Even better, *they* help determine the vision and strategy. Generally, the vision is saving the lives of patients with this condition (for us, chest pain) and lowering the cost of care.

It's important to remind everyone in the coalition to dial in the focus. We aren't trying to solve a complex problem like world hunger. Keep it practical. Think about what you see every day as it applies to this specific problem. Consider the pertinent local data and guidelines. But tap into your experience and personal knowledge. All ideas are on the table.

With a vision, you need a strategy—specific goals, objectives, and activities that populate the vision. In our coalition, the physicians embraced an ingenious method called a "consensus-written algorithm" for chest pain patients. It serves as an example not only for vision and strategy, but how to take the next crucial step: communicating the vision and strategy so effectively that the coalition grows.

Step Four:
Communicate the Change Vision

Predictably, we encountered objections as soon as we mentioned that we had an algorithm for chest pain. Good physicians will say, "Oh no, I don't follow a recipe. That's cookbook medicine." As a physician myself, I (Jeff) say the same thing.

So we went to those physicians who treat chest pain and said, "OK, given a clean slate with no systematic requirements . . . *how would you take care of a patient with chest pain?*"

The answer was always a series of, "Well, I do A. Then I do B. Then C and D and E."

We said, "Great, let's ask other esteemed physicians how they do it."

Hmm. They told us the exact same steps. In fact, the A, B, C, D, and E steps we heard for chest pain were the exact same ones I used during the episode with the senior official on Air Force One.

At this point we could say, "Look at the steps we've written down. You know what these are? A consensus-written algorithm."

This type of medical care is not a recipe or cookbook medicine. Don't think of it as an absolute dictum with consequences if you don't follow it—the same mentality we get from widget manufacturers. This is an agreed-upon guide for the 120 physicians in our EDs who treat chest pain. It's derived from a group of peers who see hundreds or thousands of chest-pain patients every year, just like you do. And if you don't follow it in every instance, that's okay. Just tell us why. We can use your input to constantly refine the algorithm.

Our methodology for chest pain quickly gained traction because physicians wrote it down *and* signed their names to it. Everyone on the medical team knew it came from the frontline staff—not from an anonymous office somewhere. Giving the physicians freedom to deviate when necessary, based on their experience with each patient, makes the algorithm more personal. Our message: *Tell us why so we can learn from you, too.*

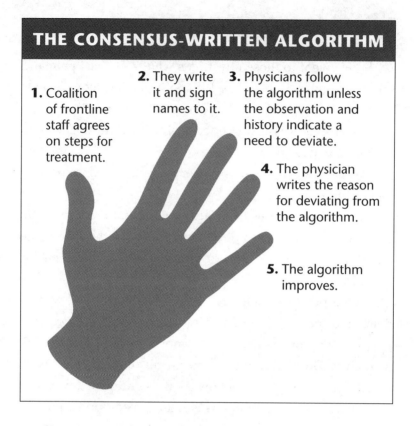

Since we implemented the chest-pain algorithm, we've found that physicians follow it more than 80 percent of the time. Someone might say, "Well, that means 20 percent of the time they're *not*." But when we examine the 20 percent, we find the reason for deviation is almost always because of individual patient variation. The patient has an arrhythmia or some other factor that follows an alternate route on the algorithm.

We were empowering the staff to individualize patient care, which fell right into the crosshairs of our vision. It added immeasurable energy to the entire cycle of transformation.

Step Five:
Empower Employees for Broad-based Action

You hear it whenever a new idea is implemented—especially after it's embraced as a success: "Oh, I had that idea eight years ago." You know what? They probably did. Which points to the fact that big systems that have been around for more than a hundred years, like those in healthcare, are replete with change barriers.

This is why the fifth step calls for team members to actively participate. To do that, we first must identify barriers that prevent a vision and strategy (like an algorithm to treat chest pain) from seeing the light of day. The barrier must be clear to everyone in the coalition. Most likely, you won't overcome the obstacle in a day or a week. But being aware of the barrier and working to remove it will allow you to keep progressing rather than turning the other way or ignoring it. If you do that, the barrier will appear later and disrupt anything you've accomplished.

One of the barriers we identified in chest pain is the amount of metrics we have to wrestle with in every case. The bookkeeping of these 50 or 100 measures often feels like a quagmire, which isn't necessarily the best use of our time when a sick patient needs attention. Our coalition took the barrier of metrics head-on by simplifying all of them into three key decision points, or performance measures:

1. Am I going to keep this patient or release this patient and follow up with care?
2. Using the stratification tool known as the HEART Score (History, EKG, Age, Risk Factors, Troponin), is this patient a high risk, intermediate risk, or low risk for heart attack in the next 45 days? (The key performance measure isn't how many patients fall into each segment. It's simply "did you use the stratification tool?")

3. How many chest-pain patients who are safely discharged from the ED are given an appointment to follow up within 72 hours—and actually return for that follow-up?

By empowering employees broadly to take action and to make adjustments as necessary, the algorithm and the key performance measures spread organically into all eight of our emergency departments.

Step Six:
Generate Short-term Wins

One of the outgrowths of being in an evidence-minded environment like healthcare is a feeling you're always in Missouri—the "show me" state. You will always have the doubting Thomases who won't change until you present irrefutable evidence. However, once you have proof, even the naysayers turn into true believers.

With our chest-pain project, we chose a hospital with about 300 beds. They see about 100,000 patients a year in their emergency department, so it's a busy place. They also had two of the champions from our coalition practicing there. During the two-month pilot, the ED physicians followed the consensus-written algorithm while seeing 400 patients. It so happened that a doctor was about to discharge the second patient in the pilot because he considered her low risk, but then he decided to follow the algorithm just in case. When he did the second troponin blood test, it turned out positive. That step in the algorithm saved the patient's life.

We could not have imagined a more effective short-term win.

The medical team shared the story and the results (data supporting the effort) from the pilot back to the coalition, to the emergency physicians, and to the system-wide group of cardiologists, hospital clinicians, and all the different stakeholders. People throughout the system, even doubters, began to advocate for the chest-pain algorithm.

Step Seven:
Consolidate Gains and Produce More Change

In a relatively short period of time, the methodology in the ED convinced physicians to discharge far more patients than previously, with confidence. None of those patients had a recurring episode within 30 days. So while lives were still being saved, costs were being cut, too.

Patients became ambassadors in the community, and physicians in the ED became champions for change within the hospitals. The message being spread was: This new algorithm doesn't make your job harder; it makes it better—for you and especially for the patient. That's what healthcare is supposed to be all about, right?

You can see at this stage how something as black and white and skeletal as an algorithm can gradually grow flesh, motion, and a life all its own. We're continually gathering input from medical staff, feeding the key measures into the cycle, holding the teams accountable, learning from other hospitals, and adding fuel to the momentum. It's kind of like a sourdough starter that never stops building and maturing, whether it's a year old or 150 years old. As long as you keep it nourished, it will sustain itself.

Step Eight:
Anchor the New Approach into the Culture

As you arrive at step eight, it's easy to take a deep breath and say, "All right. We're crossing the finish line." But this is the wrong time to coast. Strategies for long-term change often break down right here. Using the sourdough analogy: stop feeding it ... and it dies. But if you keep the nourishment coming, it just gets better. The culture continues to grow and flourish.

An example: Our teams have accepted the chest-pain methodology so fully that they've embedded the HEART score into the electronic medical record. Yes, the dreaded EMR is part of the culture change, too. Those who once considered the data-centric EMR a nemesis to their work now have a reason to embrace it.

Before we started this chest-pain project, we hadn't heard of anyone within healthcare utilizing the eight-step change process. It's always been rapid-cycle improvements, PI projects, lean processes, and quick wins. Real transformation hasn't happened. We're now several years into our change and it's become ingrained in the lifestyle. We meet new residents for the first time and start to describe the chest-pain methodology, and they'll say, "Oh yeah, of course. That's been around here for decades, hasn't it?" Or, we receive messages from physicians who go to other hospitals and ask, "Hey, can you send me the algorithm? We don't use it here, and it's hard to work without it."

ANATOMY OF CHEST PAIN RESPONSE IN THE ER		
CHEST PAIN VISIT	PRE-TRANSFORMATION	POST-TRANSFORMATION
Chest Pain Patients Per Month	4,000	4,000
Discharged	25%	59%
Admitted	25%	10%
Held for Observation	50%	31%

That's when you know you've changed the culture. The algorithm is fully implemented and into the sustain phase, you're generating wins, and the ambassadors are multiplying. Nothing is etched in stone or commanded from the top down. The cycle is in constant motion, with everyone moving it forward, and that's why it works. This is innovation in its truest sense.

The Key to Innovation Doesn't *Have* to be Disruptive

We've become fascinated with innovation both inside and outside healthcare. It's given us a gig economy, crowd sourcing, and technology we never dreamed of fifteen years ago. Authors and speakers are making fortunes on the subject of disruptive innovation. But innovation doesn't require a giant investment or massive overhauls.

Innovation can be a new idea. It can start with three people in the corner, with no new capital, no new tech, and no new hires. We're changing a culture by appealing to the hearts, heads, and hands of the people who entered healthcare for the purpose of helping others.

The Hearts: With doctors and nurses, the primary appeal is to the heart. This is the *why* of their work. They want to do what's best for the patient. What could be more appealing from the chest-pain project than the potential to save lives?

The Heads: From there we appeal to the thought process, or *what* the doctors and nurses will be doing with the methodology. We promise this isn't a recipe; it's an agreed-upon method you and your peers have come up with.

The Hands: And then we appeal to the hands, taking the words and guidance of the methodology and showing *how* to put it into action. We've heard doctors say, "I came to a key decision point and wasn't sure which way to go... so I went to the algorithm."

It would be much simpler if we could change a culture through baptism—or even through Six Sigma or lean production strategies. But cultures don't change that way. As we saw with something as specific as a chest-pain project, *experience* changes a culture.

> This type of medical care is not a recipe or cookbook medicine.

You can compare this project, or any project like it, to a pot of water over a campfire. When you heat the water from the bottom, you'll first see little bubbles rising around the edges. A minute later you'll see those little bubbles gathering to form bigger bubbles... until you have a full boil. The entire pot of water undergoes massive change, and yet the whole process started quietly. Now imagine if we'd gone into our project with limited patience, mandates, and a few new fancy tools—the rapid-change approach. We would have gone into it as if trying to heat the pot of water with a blowtorch, from the top down. You eventually have some warm water on the surface, but scoop it out and you find all the water underneath is unchanged. You're back to square one. The cycle only moves forward if the energy comes from within.

The Lancet Turns Up the Heat

We mentioned in chapter one that *The Lancet* published our methodology for chest pain, as well as the quantified money and lives saved. The article came out as we were developing this book. The recognition of our work added momentum to the change effort because it comes from such a highly respected group of peers. In *The Lancet*'s article we explained the problem that thousands of medical personnel know all too well: that misdiagnoses of chest pain in emergency departments cost lives, while low-risk patients being overtested and overadmitted costs money.

The Lancet described our vision to establish what we would eventually call the AdventHealth Clinical Transformation (ACT) method. Among our first steps were investigating change management ideas and digging into projects launched in the Netherlands and eighteen tertiary referral centers in the US. This background and our own experiences caring for patients led us to use the HEART Score (History, EKG, Age, Risk factors, and Troponin) as a baseline to differentiate patients as either low risk or high risk. In turn, that's what led to changes so radical that they can only be called "transformative" (we'll share specifics throughout the book).

> Physician behavior can be changed and sustained by inviting them into the ongoing process.

But the scores themselves aren't the transformation. The most telling points in *The Lancet* article emphasize the buy-in we received from a traditionally reluctant group of practitioners. After seeing the results from our two-month pilot, cardiologists and emergency medicine physicians from our healthcare system unanimously approved the implementation of our ACT algorithm. You read that right: we received *unanimous* approval, which is almost unheard of. Only six months after the pilot, our ACT algorithm was fully implemented system-wide. When we say "our" algorithm, we mean the algorithm credited to a whole team of frontline leaders (giving credit is an important part of transformation, which we'll explain later in detail).

In other words, as the paper says, we proved in the first pilot that physician behavior can be changed and sustained by inviting them into the ongoing process. And that's how permanent change happens—by heating the pot of water from deep inside.

How Serious Are You?

This leads us to the critical moment of truth for healthcare leaders. Here we have the method, the example, and the ongoing results from one clinical problem—chest pain. We've saved lives and money. We have believers and a changed culture. So the question lingering in the air is this: If we present you with a proven path for transformation, will you be willing to take it?

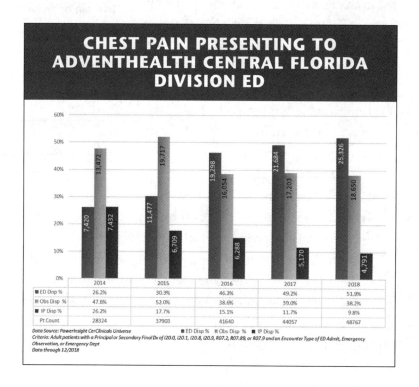

KEY POINTS FROM CHAPTER FOUR

- **Your first breakthrough.** The challenge—and the blessing—in transforming healthcare is to shatter the status quo.

- **Confessing a big problem.** Too many patients with chest pain are unnecessarily admitted. This issue was the first to be tackled as we began our quest to transform healthcare.

- **Chest pain in emergency departments.** The key question: is it safe to admit, hold for observation, or discharge? Our algorithm supplied the tools the front line needed to make an informed decision.

- **Eight change management principles.** Implemented for the first time in healthcare, these principles led us to transform the way we treat patients with chest pain.

- **The HEART Score.** It's easy to remember, easy to use, and changes the game.

- **Long-term benefits.** Our plan, or "algorithm," leads to constant improvements in care. Consider using our template to create algorithms of your own.

- **Help peers accept the methodology.** As you successfully make changes using the algorithm, be sure to document your successes and publish them for the benefit of the healthcare community, just as we did when we published our article in *The Lancet* about our results with chest pain.

- **Encourage peers to embrace the methodology.** We presented our findings to cardiologists and emergency department physicians who unanimously approved the changes, which were then implemented system-wide. You can do the same.

REFLECTIONS

- Look at the area of care you identified at the end of chapter three. Write a brief summary of what makes that area an urgent cause for change.
- Write down the names of the 5–10 people who:
    1. would champion the journey;
    2. would collaborate well on a team to discuss new approaches to the care mentioned above;
    3. are able to think creatively;
    4. would be influential at the front lines and in the front offices.

CHAPTER 5

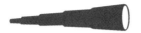

Turning Our Model on Its Head

People, Processes, Technology

Whenever people hear that I (Jeff) spent more than 16 years as the physician for the president and senior officials, they ask, "What was your favorite part about the job?" Well, I supplied medical support in the White House, but also wherever the president traveled in the US and around the world. So my answer to the question is, "The travel." The inevitable follow-up question is, "What's the worst part of the job?" And my answer is, "The travel."

During those years I had the opportunity to go to about ninety countries, seeing remarkable sights and experiencing unique cultures. And in those ninety countries I would evaluate the healthcare infrastructures—including access to emergency care right down to the minute details. You don't realize the significance of those details until there's an unforeseen medical event. Nowhere did those details become more profound in importance than in China, or Beijing, to be exact.

I took my first swing through China supporting President Clinton in June 1998. Beijing fascinated me—the food, the architecture, and the millions of people riding bicycles around the Forbidden City. The country had been cloaked in privacy for generations, leaving rough artwork to give us the best renditions of life there. Seeing it with my own eyes was like pulling back the curtain and watching a very different culture unfold on a stage.

It turns out, those first glimpses did not reveal key differences behind the scenes where key decisions are made. I would discover a few of them on a future visit.

Ten years later I returned to Beijing as part of the pre-advance team for President Bush, who would be attending the opening and closing ceremonies of the 2008 Summer Olympics. The pre-advance team goes out a couple of months early to explore where the venues are, how to expediently get around, and what barriers might be in the way. You work with the local security and healthcare officials on an emergency plan in case something goes terribly wrong, no matter how unlikely it seems.

Doing this type of planning in a country so culturally and politically disparate from your own pits you against strong cultural standards. You're on someone else's turf, and even though you notice things that need to be changed, you have to be careful when you speak up. It's almost like trying to alter long-held protocols in our own healthcare system—the barriers are rigid and rampant. In Beijing we didn't want to overhaul the system; we only needed a reasonable emergency plan. If only we could break those barriers.

Our hosts in Beijing were initially surprised to hear we didn't need to use the prettiest hospital in case of an emergency. We'd learned from previous travel to choose the hospital that sees the most trauma cases. Sometimes that causes grief with the local officials. They often want to use an opportunity like this to show the visitors their best side, which for a hospital means the one with the best cafeteria or where the grandmother of a top official was given exceptional care. But all we want to know is which one treats the most knife and gunshot wounds.

Turns out, the hospital we chose isn't situated next to the shiny new Olympic venues—the Bird's Nest or the Ice Cube or the Olympic Village—but is near Tiananmen Square, about ten miles away. There at the hospital, our medical team asked where a trauma patient would enter, who would staff the emergency unit, and for the step-by-step guidelines of how the patient would theoretically be treated. In my role, you take special note of the decontamination procedures, the trauma stabilization—the gritty stuff you hope to never need. Regardless, you have to plan for the worst.

> Using our methodology, you may not cure every patient, but you will provide whole-person healing for each and every patient.

The people showing us around were reluctant to answer my questions about trauma care. They only wanted to show me their new VIP wing, which looked like a rooftop suite at the Ritz-Carlton. Even the embassy doctor kept ushering my attention to the creature comforts. I'd traveled enough and seen some swank places, so none of this impressed me. A patient in an emergency won't be ordering filet mignon from a recliner. After politely following my hosts around for a bit, I finally told them, "Look, this is the bottom line: If an individual gets shot or stabbed, we have to keep the blood in the body and get them to definitive care. And then your trauma team needs to be here to continue the care."

The whole scene I described seemed completely foreign to them. Their idea of a trauma team is one that sits at home and, if they're summoned, comes in to do their jobs. When I pressed the issue, they actually said, "There will not be a gunshot wound. There will not be a stabbing. *It will not happen here.*"

They had expectations and procedures, which were rooted partly in old traditions but also in the desire to assert a safe appearance to people visiting from afar. There's a fine line in diplomacy where you either accept the standards of a culture or you speak up. So I said, "That's great to know. But we need a plan in place anyway."

After some back and forth, the medical officials placated me and said they'd have two trauma teams in place, taking alternating shifts. We worked out the transportation aspect, point of entry, supplies . . . the specifics of care just in case the unthinkable happened.

In August we arrived with Air Force One, the support plane, the media plane, and the president and his entourage. The night of the opening ceremony went without incident. The next morning, while everyone was still abuzz about the incredible display the night before, the family of a US Olympic coach (his wife, father-in-law, and mother-in-law) were taking in the views from a tower near Tiananmen Square . . . when a man pulled a knife and stabbed the in-laws. The father-in-law died. The mother-in-law suffered abdominal wounds and was bleeding badly. The local emergency medical team kept the blood in her body and transported her to the trauma center, which was fully staffed. Every person on the trauma team, from the first points of contact in the public square to the hospital's emergency department, followed the steps we had set up in the trauma plan two months earlier.

The mother-in-law's life was saved.

You Choose: The Protocol or the Patient

Had our advance medical team in Beijing followed the protocols of the hospital and government officials, had we acquiesced to their long-held local beliefs about the incidence of trauma, two people would have died that day in Tiananmen Square. So what does this story have to do with transforming healthcare in the US? We have our own sacred cows and long-standing mindsets. And many of them have to be removed if we're going to do what's best for the current and future patient.

In China, we found the conventional approach to healthcare is to believe "it will never happen here." That mindset is a barrier to change. In our system, the conventional approach is to go immediately to the technology and data to direct our medical care. And our reliance on tech and data has become a barrier to transforming healthcare.

Give credit to the team in Beijing. Once we explained what we needed to do, why we needed to do it, and how we'd do it, they understood and made necessary changes. Also important was that we listened to them describe the key barriers to those changes. Mostly they said, "It's bureaucratic. If we do this, it will appear as if we're expecting a tragedy."

Through our conversation we allowed them to identify the barriers, and then we all discreetly worked through them. If we hadn't, their deeply anchored modus operandi could very well have kept a patient from receiving lifesaving care.

Now think of how technology and data are becoming the be-all, end-all in our healthcare. There's no question technology helps us make diagnoses, transmit information, and properly treat patients. However, when we build healthcare around technology and data, we become as restricted as the person in another country who will not consider a plan for trauma. The very protocols we heavily depend on overwhelm our greatest assets in making proper medical decisions. Those greatest assets? Practice, experience, personal expertise, observation . . . and, at the top, the physician-patient relationship.

The Most Important Fifteen Minutes

It's helpful to frequently think of the patient sitting on the exam table or attempting to sit in a chair as the doctor enters the room. This scenario happens thousands of times every day—different conditions, of course, but the general setting is easy to picture. Let's say the patient in this case is grimacing and they're positioned a little bit sideways. The experienced physician walks in, looks at the patient, asks a couple of questions, and says, "Oh, you have a thrombosed hemorrhoid."

Well, the doctor could and really *should* make it so simple. But the real-life requirements and expectations in today's healthcare don't always allow it.

Doctors typically have exactly fifteen minutes to see a patient. During that time, they need to find out what's wrong and come up with a plan for treatment. At least eight or ten of those minutes are burned as the doctor fills out the checklist on a computer or tablet. As a patient, you're sitting there partly naked in a gown with no back to it. You don't feel well. You're concerned to some degree about your health. The person you trust to provide the best care is in the room with you. But instead of conversing, you have to sit and watch him or her poke a screen for the majority of your time together. It's worse than trying to talk with a friend over lunch while they text some *other* friend—who, it appears, is more important than you.

The patient is wondering, "What could be more important than me right now?"

Let's say the doctor finally looks up from the computer and says, "I'm sorry to tell you, but . . ."

Does the patient feel like the center of attention? Undoubtedly, patients often leave doctors' offices wondering if they really received the best care possible, or if they simply received the most convenient care based on the output of a computer program.

How much better would it be if we spent fourteen of those fifteen minutes talking with the patient? Healthcare would be perceived completely different than it is today. There would be more trust, more optimism, and legitimate mind-body-spirit healing.

Modern Healthcare, Simplified

In the first week of medical school, we learned three things:

- One, listen to your patient and they'll tell you what's wrong.
- Two, don't be overenamored or too dependent on technology.
- And three, give every patient something for their time of need. Sometimes that will be a medication. Other times it might be a procedure. And then there are times when they'll need a hand to hold, a shoulder for comfort, or a listening ear.

It's pretty simple, really. The patient wants to be assured of a proper diagnosis. So does the medical team. From there you can formulate a plan for healing. And, as a doctor, almost everything necessary is right there in front of you—the patient can tell you.

The three tenets we learned in medical school still hold true. The fact is, a patient's history tells you 80 percent of what you need to know. The physical evidence tells you 10–15 percent. And then the diagnostics, the lab, the imaging, the fancy technology adds maybe 5–10 percent to your decision making. With that, you can sketch out a basic pyramid for ideal healthcare.

People provide the deep and strong base: 80 percent.
Physical evidence holds the middle part of the pyramid together: 10–15 percent.
Technology adds the little extra up top: 5–10 percent.

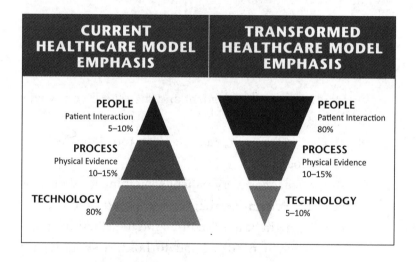

Gathering data from a distant information system is not the best or most direct way to treat the patient in the room. However, it's very easy and oftentimes required to be sidetracked with a computer readout or a scan or a test (the test itself might be necessary or . . . might not). All of which often leads to unintentionally ignoring the patient, let alone attempting to relate to their condition.

We've literally turned the most logical and effective pyramid of care upside down. Technology dominates. Artificial intelligence is also upon us. These are fantastic tools. In the hands of doctors, they can effectively supplement observations and the relationship with the patient. They're hugely beneficial, but our total reliance on them has led to what we now consider "modern healthcare."

And modern healthcare—the pyramid with technology anchoring everything—has given us high costs, in terms of both money and lives.

The only way we'll move out of this storm is to pull up the anchor that's holding us back, just as the advance medical team in China had to pry the professionals from their anchor. It's a culture change. Technology won't make it happen. People will.

Generation Next

Watch the commercials for hospitals. Look at the promotional materials. The pretty facilities and leading-edge technology take the starring roles because they make the most immediate impressions. We admit that an algorithm for chest pain or sepsis will probably not make the cut into a TV ad. Game changing? Yes. Visually stunning? No.

However, when we gather input from doctors and nurses across our system, representing every medical department and at least four generations, not once have we been asked to add more technology or another tower into our methodology—let alone lead with it. The medical teams are telling us they'd rather start with a HEART Score than a CT scan. They want to provide personalized care instead of tech-centric care. This feedback is telling, because all you need to do is watch how often your phone updates by itself to see that changing technology is far easier than changing people. But the focal point of healthcare isn't a phone or a widget.

A COMPARISON OF CHEST PAIN RESPONSES

CURRENT RESPONSE TO CHEST PAIN	TRANSFORMED RESPONSE TO CHEST PAIN
Order a CT scan.	Ask questions.
Hold patient for costly test results and further observation.	Perform a HEART score: History, EKG, Age, Risk Factors, Troponin.
Higher probability of admitting the patient before knowing if it's necessary.	Higher probability of releasing the patient with follow-up scheduled.

There are at least three clear reasons why physicians and nurses who have used our patient-first algorithms believe in them and *want* them:

1. They work. We've proven this with every algorithm. Lives are being saved.
2. Medical teams like patient-specific algorithms because they are not business models. Nowhere in our original charge to transform our healthcare did a conversation come up about hospital profits. It just so happens, however, that the success of these algorithms also translates to better overall business—costs are saved and beds are available for patients with more serious conditions.
3. Although the word "algorithm" sounds academic and impersonal, it is the polar opposite. Everything about the algorithms, which, remember, are developed and nuanced by the medical teams, points to interactions

with the patient. This personal approach also bridges the gap between generational physicians—the silent generation, baby boomers, Generation Xers, and millennials. It bridges the language gap between physicians and administrators. The algorithms are conduits from people to people.

Using our methodology, you may not cure every patient, but you *will* provide whole-person healing for each and every patient. Because the healthcare we all want (better diagnoses and better outcomes) comes when information is woven into relationships. Not just any information—*helpful* information. Where we find helpful information and how we use it . . . that's another key to transforming healthcare.

KEY POINTS FROM CHAPTER FIVE

- **Holding onto old protocols.** It can be difficult to let go of old protocols we are familiar with, but our unwillingness to change can cost people lives.

- **Data and tech.** Data and tech have become the "old protocols" in the US healthcare system, where the conventional approach is to go immediately to technology and data to direct our medical care. Our reliance on tech and data has become a barrier to transforming healthcare.

- **First med-school lessons.** Listen to the patient. Don't rely on technology to answer the question. Give our patients something in their time of need.

- **The best medical model.** Technology and data play a supporting, not a lead, role in practice. When technology anchors everything, we get high costs in both lives and money.

- **Algorithms work.** Medical teams want to provide personalized care rather than tech-centric care. Staff-driven plans for care make believers of everyone who uses them.

REFLECTIONS

- In what ways can your champions better work patient interaction into care (history, observation, etc.)?

- How could those elements be rolled into an easy-to-follow algorithm—one that any healthcare worker could use?

- How can your champions integrate that information?

CHAPTER 6

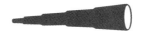

Our Most Powerful Tool

You Don't Need a Manual to Use Synthetical Thinking

The mere thought of baseball cards brings back a flood of childhood memories for me (Jeff). I can still feel what it's like to pull apart the wrapper on a pack of cards and then to chew the thin strip of bubble gum that would lose its flavor before I could even see which players were among the small stack of ten cards. If you collected baseball cards, you know what I'm talking about. You'd quickly flip through the cards to look at the pictures and names of the players . . . and then you'd turn them over one by one and spend part of the afternoon looking at the good stuff: the statistics on the back.

In sports, and especially baseball, statistics mean information. Fans are enamored with statistics because you can compare the numbers from player to player, no matter if those players are modern-day rivals or were active fifty years apart from each other. Statistics transcend time. They allow us to place perceived value on players. They make us feel smarter. Some of the numbers in baseball are ethereal: 755 (the number of home runs Hank Aaron hit), 4,256 (the number of hits for all-time leader Pete Rose), a .300 hitter is better than a .250 hitter, 300 strikeouts means you must be a great pitcher.

It's funny because if you mention any of these statistics to someone from the UK, you'll get a blank stare. The numbers are meaningless. Non-baseball fans just want to know, "Who won?" In fact, in the UK where cricket is king, you keep loads of statistics for the purpose of proving the result at the end of the game . . . most times, a draw!

So, although statistics give us benchmarks to compare players and analyze performances, the truth is, they aren't as helpful at predicting or determining outcomes as we might think. Gaudy statistics can look good on a player profile, but if they don't help the team win then you have to wonder what difference they really make. The value of statistics is providing us easy-to-use information to compare, debate, and to affix to memories.

Statistics in sports epitomize the use of *analytical thinking*. In healthcare, we've been following a very similar way of thinking. And it isn't the best use of our minds.

Five Types of Thinking (And the One in All of Us)

In the early 1980s, back when the Boston Red Sox were still pilloried for their inability to win a baseball world championship, Doctors Allen F. Harrison and Robert M. Bramson released a book entitled *The Art of Thinking*. They called it "the classic guide to increasing brain power." The book includes self-assessments so readers can categorize themselves into one of five types of thinkers:

The Pragmatist is always looking for the quickest route to a positive result. Cut corners. Justify decisions along the way. If something works, just make it happen.

The Idealist takes all the time and energy necessary to make the best decision possible, even if the hoped-for result is out of reach. Maybe you can get there next time.

The Realist is only interested in facts and feedback from the few people thought to be experts. No matter how you cut it, the results are predictable.

This takes us to the other two types of thinkers: one who typifies where we are in healthcare, and one who exemplifies where we *want* to be.

The Analyst is the category where most Americans tend to lean and which dominates how we think (or are directed to think) in healthcare. Decisions are to be based solely on data and scientific solutions. Analysis paints a picture of the evidence-based healthcare model that so many systems believe in. Yet it does not necessarily describe the actual work of the best practitioners as referenced in the study at Harvard in chapter 4. This ideal is to look at an isolated step and scrutinize the individual step.

And this takes us to the type of thinker who will literally transform healthcare:

The Synthetical Thinker is harder to find. Or so it seems. This person wants to change the status quo by considering input from a wide variety of sources. They recognize the value of concrete data and abstract information—without overvaluing the former. They value expert opinions and grassroots ideas. Intuition and experience. Environmental factors and history. Studies and firsthand knowledge. The goal is not to find an easy answer or a formulaic solution, but rather to use every resource available to reach the optimum outcome.

The analysts are all around us. They drive the healthcare system with lean processes, best practices, and data-centric protocols. Whether we know it or not, most of us have been groomed into the analyst group.

But the synthetical thinkers are all around us, too. This type of thinking attracted the majority of us into healthcare in the first place. It enables us to put disparate ideas together into one coherent plan. You might not know it from the way your work has changed, but *the synthetical thinker is none other than you.*

Yes, *you* are the synthetical thinker. Which means *you* are equipped to transform the way we care for patients wherever you're doing it.

FIVE TYPES OF THINKING IN HEALTHCARE	
01	**ANALYTICAL** Lean processes. "What's the most efficient way to get it done?"
02	**PRAGMATIC** Do it. "Let's get this done as quickly as possible and move on."
03	**IDEALISTIC** Whatever it takes. "Take your time. Reach for ideal outcomes."
04	**REALISTIC** Cut to the chase. "Before we start, what do we know for sure?"
05	**SYNTHETICAL** All types of input are on the table. "Everyone be flexible."

For Those Who Think Statistics Don't Lie . . .

Statistics look as valuable and proper in medical journals as they do on baseball cards. In the same respect, those statistics don't necessarily have anything to do with the unique situation literally at hand, at this very moment. In baseball, a batting average doesn't tell you how the player performs in cold weather or how well he moves his teammates along from one base to the next. The stats on a baseball card don't reflect fielding range or the strength of a throwing arm. Traditional analysis in sports doesn't capture leadership qualities or the willingness of a player to actually *sacrifice* his or her statistics for the good of the team at any given moment.

Despite the very names of some baseball statistics ("wins" for a pitcher or "wins above replacement" for any position), a player with lofty numbers doesn't literally *win* games. Teams do. Statistics are only part of a much larger equation—an equation that expands beyond analysis.

You can make the same correlation to healthcare. Taking care of a patient is often complex. It requires listening, looking, and feeling. Patient history is a critical factor, as is your own experience as a physician. An isolated set of metrics is no more effective for the care of the patient than a personal batting average is for the success of the team. Could it be helpful? Yes . . . maybe . . . hard to say. We can't afford those types of answers in healthcare.

One metric that frequently comes up in the front offices of hospitals is the number of patient readmissions within thirty days. A straight analysis of the readmission statistics might seem to tell us, "If the number is low, then we must be healing patients at a positive rate, because they aren't coming back. That's good." Are you sure about that? Or could it be that some patients didn't come back because they had a bad experience? Maybe some patients died. Analytical thinking takes none of those possibilities into account.

Physicians vs. Statisticians

Baseball teams have become more astute about keeping statistics. The baseball card is for fans only. Every team now has hosts of personnel who chart every pitch, every swing, and every conceivable pitcher-hitter matchup. They use 3D Doppler radar systems to track spin rates of pitches, loft angles of fly balls, and a flurry of information that wasn't available until the past ten years. The data is filtered, studied, and summarized for the coaching staffs to use while they make game-day decisions. But coaches aren't required to use the data. Their decisions are based on a host of factors—including the situation and personal intuition.

The additional data has, if anything, fueled more synthetical thinking. And it works.

But imagine if the manager and his coaches were tasked with inputting all of the data themselves. What if they weren't really there to make decisions, but rather they were simply conduits or deliverers of decisions found on a computer screen? It's silly to even think of making important choices that way. However, that's a pretty accurate analogy of how physicians are now told to do their work.

The EMR in the past couple of decades has risen in importance to where it directs decisions in the administrative offices and also in the patient rooms. It's a financial record, a medical record, a list of protocols and processes, and in some respects the EMR is now the fulcrum in what we would loosely call "the relationship with our patient."

The reality is this: many doctors say the EMR has caused paralysis by analysis . . . which has contributed to burnout.

A consortium of the Massachusetts Medical Society, Massachusetts Health and Hospital Association, and Harvard published research indicating burnout among more than 40 percent of physicians.[12] The American Medical Association writes that the paper "illustrates the growing recognition that an energized, engaged, and resilient workforce is essential to achieving national health goals." It goes on to say, "Mounting obstacles to patient care contribute to emotional fatigue, depersonalization, and loss of enthusiasm among physicians." Almost 60 percent of physicians pointed to "too many bureaucratic tasks" as the leading cause of burnout—specifically, excess processing of charts and paperwork.

So, by asking physicians to be recordkeepers, we now have less personalized care than ever and a higher instance of burnout. Key measures in the most important areas of healthcare—patient satisfaction and employee satisfaction—are sluggish at best. Patient satisfaction scores are attributed to the doctor but in reality reflect the success or failure of the system as a whole. The system attributes a poor score to a physician who has many demands that compete for time spent with the patient. It's obvious that physicians and nurses don't want to be data input analysts. When it comes to caring for patients, they want to be synthesists, whether they've heard the word or not. Put it this way: we don't know anyone in our healthcare system who learned to practice medicine for the love of statistics.

A Cloud with All the Healthcare Answers

In the universe of technology, the cloud is a place in the ether where information is stored and accessed as needed. We also have a cloud available for healthcare decisions. It combines verbal history, family history, firsthand observation, physician experiences, environmental factors, perhaps a blood test or imaging . . . everything about a patient is uploaded to a place where it's blended together and then delivered back to the bedside.

The kind of cloud we describe here is *not* an EMR. This cloud is the physician himself or herself. With the assistance of data, a doctor can and *should* be enabled to make wholistic health decisions based on know-how—and using an algorithm. In totality, *this cloud is synthetical thinking*. And it is extraordinarily powerful.

The best chefs give us great illustrations of synthetical thinking. You can give a lasagna recipe to a chef and instruct her to stick to it, word by word, from start to finish. She'll probably come out to the table with a decent plate of lasagna. But it isn't her *best* version of the dish, the one she learned from watching her grandmother, then training in culinary school, and gaining experience in restaurants around the world, where she developed amazing flavor profiles. This chef is at her best when you say, "Here are some top-shelf ingredients and cooking tools . . . go ahead and make your best lasagna." She looks, she smells, she samples, and brings everything together. Out of that comes an amazing dish that you would never experience anywhere else. When you ask for *her* secret ingredients (and this is true of most chefs), she says, "The most important ingredients are the time and passion I put into each dish."

The same principles apply to healthcare. If you look only at data, turn it into a process, and tell the doctors and nurses on your team, "OK, this is the way we're going to treat patients, period," the results won't be great. Doctors will be pressed for time. They'll forget their passion for medicine. The process will be expensive. And people won't enjoy healthy lives as they should.

Our best doctors use the exact words of the best chefs: "I don't follow a recipe." That's what we want them to say. However, there *are* some useful steps. Ask ten chefs how to make a certain dish and all ten will mention the same basic ingredients. They'll use their own twists during the preparation, depending on factors like environment and the guests. But for the most part, the framework of the dish is the same from chef to chef.

That's what we've done with our algorithms. Every doctor will use the same eight steps to care for a specific health situation. We capture those steps in the algorithm so physicians can use it while also synthetically thinking through the nuances for each specific patient. They adjust the algorithm to suit the situation.

> In our work, success is helping patients heal more completely and live healthier, longer lives.

But let's say an adjustment to the algorithm makes it better. Then what? I mean, if your Italian great-aunt makes a dish like you've never tasted and she doesn't write down her method, then it's lost forever when she can no longer cook. You want her to write it down—or you want to do it with her—so you have the method to pass on to other generations. The dish will never taste exactly the same as hers—she had a special touch and made it a little bit different depending on what she saw, smelled, and felt. But for the most part she followed the same "algorithm." And from that, with your own little adjustments, you can still make a pretty spectacular meal.

That's how doctors and nurses create a pathway for transformed healthcare. You use the guidelines and your own observations. Your coalition that provides the care every day (the "culinary team in the kitchen") creates an algorithm and writes it down. Most people on your medical team will follow it because of the influence of the coalition. But you give them permission to deviate whenever it's best to do so for the patient. Again, it's synthetical thinking rather than analytical thinking.

INGREDIENTS OF SYNTHETICAL THINKING

- Firsthand observation
- Patient's verbal history
- Patient's family history
- Physician experiences
- Environmental factors
- Blood test or imaging
- Supporting data

Your Most Critical Question

We should always be asking, "What's the meaning of success in our work?" In baseball, the sport once fastened to the statistics found on baseball cards has progressed. You hear the word "analytics" used quite often in the sport, but the best decision makers are actually using synthetical thinking. Millennials in front offices are rallying together all the input available to evaluate player performances and team chemistry. The new practice has transformed some losing franchises into championship contenders, because everyone from the field to the front office realizes that statistics are not the ultimate goal in baseball, cricket, or in any sport. It's winning.

In our work, success is helping patients heal more completely and live healthier, longer lives. We earn victories one patient at a time. And as more patients live better than ever, we'll transform healthcare into a winning culture. Come on, if baseball can use synthetical thinking to generate wins, then we can do the same in healthcare.

KEY POINTS FROM CHAPTER SIX

- **Number-one reason for physician burnout.** Research shows that almost 60 percent of physicians pointed to "too many bureaucratic tasks" as the leading cause of burnout—specifically, excess processing of charts and paperwork. Our reliance on feeding data into electronic medical records is costing us time, money, and good people.

- **The five types of thinking.** Some authors categorize people into one of five types of thinkers. You're either a pragmatist, an idealist, a realist, an analyst, or a synthetical thinker.

- **The power of "synthetical thinking."** In the universe of technology, the cloud is a place in the ether where information is stored and accessed as needed. The physician should be seen as our "cloud" of expertise, using observation, information, experience, and relationships to treat each patient.

- **Doctors are like chefs.** Our best doctors use the exact words of the best chefs: "I don't follow a recipe." Give them the tools and ingredients and trust them to work their craft.

REFLECTIONS

- Write down the meaning of "success" in your care for a patient.
- What type of thinker are you, honestly?
- What components of synthetical thinking are currently missing from your team's work, and how can you work them into patient care?

CHAPTER 7

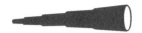

Doing Is Believing

The Cycle of Transformation in Real Life

Before entering the medical field, I (Danny) worked in private law enforcement. For a number of years, I led a group that specialized in investigative work for major theme parks. You're probably thinking, "Oh, I bet you have some interesting stories." Yes, we could have been the subject of a good reality-television show. Among all the stories, however, one always stands out to me. It provides a vivid example of how people in the trenches can make dramatic impact on the big-picture work of any organization.

So it's midmorning at one of the parks when I get a call from a store clerk. A guest has just used a traveler's check to pay for some souvenirs—a common type of transaction in the 1990s when traveler's checks are said to be convenient and safe to use anywhere in the world. With any type of currency, however, retailers have to be extra cautious where large crowds of people are making clusters of transactions. Scammers view such places as opportunities to strike. Knowing this, we've trained the clerks in this park to identify the signs of a questionable exchange. They've learned a series of steps using sight, touch, and intuition to decipher legitimate currency from the possibly illegitimate. In a way, the steps are an algorithm, developed with input from the team members.

The frontline clerk has called because the check used for this particular purchase doesn't feel quite right. She reads the numbers on the check over the phone and tells me why, in her mind, it's raised a yellow flag. I take her alertness seriously enough to call the lead investigator at the company that makes the traveler's checks. He does some quick verification, comes back to the phone, and says, "Everything is fine with the bill. Don't worry about it."

Less than an hour later, we receive a call from another team member at a different store in the park. "I have this traveler's check," he says, "and something about it doesn't look right."

This time we rush over and look at the check ourselves. Sure enough, it looks "off." We again call the investigator at the check company, and he tells us what he told us a short time earlier: "Nope, it's perfectly OK."

> When everyone has a role, no matter how inconsequential the role might seem in the hierarchy of a system, it's like energy radiating to and from an entire power grid.

We can see the paper with our eyes and touch it with our hands. No matter what we're being told from a thousand miles away, we can tell something is amiss. Our good sense tells us to start tracking the person who's using the checks. At each point of purchase, we inspect the numbers. They start to run consecutively, which is odd, so we finally pull the guy into an office where federal investigators interview him.

After a few more phone calls and deeper questioning, we discover the checks are indeed bad. Actually, they're beyond bad. The checks are part of a multimillion-dollar counterfeiting ring that stretches across six or seven countries. We've initiated a major international bust.

The reality is, our investigators and the federal investigators did not uncover the scam. Neither did the investigative team at the traveler's-check company. The credit goes to the frontline clerks in the park. You know what they used to call out the crime? Synthetical thinking. They knew the warning signs. They had their hands and eyes right there at the points of transaction. What did *my* team do in our leadership role? We gave the frontline people the proper steps to follow. We empowered them to mentally gather input and interpret it. And we listened to them.

The Power Up Front

In retail, you'd be foolish to ignore the people who are in direct contact with the customers. Or think of a farmer who isn't in the vineyard every day. If the foremen in the fields say there's a problem with pests, the farmer better listen and give them whatever the workers need to fix the issue.

It should be no different in our work. Trust the people who are taking care of the patients, day in and day out. They can identify specific problems and solve them more effectively, patient by patient, than measures developed from the distant hallowed halls of academia or "the ivory tower," so to speak. When everyone has a role, no matter how inconsequential the role might seem in the hierarchy of a system, it's like energy radiating to and from an entire power grid.

OK, so we've painted a real-life picture of a theme park. To envision transformed healthcare, and to easily apply it anywhere, let's break the image down into four phases: Design, Pilot, Implement, Sustain.

When used patiently, we've been surprised at how effectively we have transformed our care from here to there. Be warned, however, because we've also learned that if you skip a phase, you'll take ten steps back. And backward is one direction we want to avoid.

Phase 1: Design

The Front Line Initiates Change in Minutes, Hours, and Weeks

Going into our chest-pain project, we had to toss aside the old assumptions and excuses for why a change couldn't be done.

Doctors are too busy to be involved. True, their schedules have very little margin, so we have to make it convenient.

You'll never convince them to take time to talk about patient care as a group. Actually, we found the only convincing they need is the promise that their input will be put into action.

In little time we had two emergency medical physicians, two nurses, a hospitalist, and two cardiologists brainstorming together. They formed our coalition—a mix of young people with energy, and seasoned practitioners with wisdom. Everyone on the medical staff knew these people for two important qualities:

1. They're excellent at practicing medicine.
2. They're easy to work with.

How did we get them on board? We explained that our project was not for the purpose of writing a case study for a journal, nor was it an administrative exercise. Once the coalition candidates knew they'd be developing and utilizing their own methodology for patient care, and that the purpose would be to save lives and make healthcare affordable, they were eager to participate. We assured them that whatever algorithm they developed would be theirs to use and share with the frontline staff.

During the first discussion, the coalition talked about blood tests and medications. They shared thoughts about when to bring in cardiologists, when to accelerate care, and how to best identify high-, medium-, and low-risk patients. We asked questions. How would we categorize diagnostic results? When is it best to conduct a functional test versus an anatomic test of the coronary arteries?

We used all this input synthetically to reach a consensus on an algorithm for medical teams to use in real time, including the use of the stratification tool and the course of action (a procedure, a level of care, or discharge). To keep it realistic, we asked the coalition to identify the barriers they'd likely encounter when trying to use the algorithm. Together, we would either mitigate those barriers, remove them, or ask people with resources to move the big rocks out of the way.

You could sense that the coalition felt motivated, perhaps to a higher degree than we anticipated. The topic of the conversations—ideal patient care—brought them back to their ultimate purpose in healthcare, and they completed the first steps of the Design Phase quicker than anyone might have thought possible:

They agreed on a vision in a matter of minutes. This vision came together so quickly because the reason we practice medicine is our common thread. It's always on the mind. These leaders just needed an opportunity to express it.

They agreed on an algorithm within two hours. Maybe the speed it took the group to agree shouldn't be so surprising, given the fact they work with chest-pain patients all day long. They'd always known the smartest steps to take, but until now hadn't been asked to write them down.

They identified the barriers, and we had them removed in a few weeks. Having a clear vision and specific algorithm gave them a concrete reason to move heaven and earth, if that's what it took. Over time, they also found a way to use the power of the electronic medical record as a transformative factor (embedding the HEART score into the EMR).

As we said, these steps didn't take years and did not require executive summits. What this small group of frontline people developed is not a business model. It is not a pro forma. It's a method for the best way to take care of patients with chest pain.

That is, as long as the method is intentionally shepherded through the next phases.

DESIGN PHASE TIMELINE

Form Coalition	Agree on Vision	Agree on Algorithm	Identify and Remove Barriers
1 Day	30 Minutes	2–4 Hours	4–5+ Weeks

Phase 2: Pilot

Lessons Learned from Deviations

The Pilot Phase, or prototype, is where we look for those short-term wins. For our pilot with chest pain, we started at a 300-bed hospital in our system. We didn't want to simply run the pilot, leave with metrics, and use them to justify our work at another hospital. The intent is not "clinical research" or to reach a finish line. Transformation is always living and breathing. So we vowed to be transparent with whatever facts and comments came out of it—good, bad, or indifferent.

Over a two-month span, our medical team treated about 400 chest-pain patients. The team closely used the algorithm in about 80 percent of those cases and gave us feedback from those experiences. Perhaps more interesting were the lessons we learned from the 20 percent where the teams *didn't* follow the algorithm as written. The deviations, even slight, provided valuable insight to improve the methodology. Eighty percent of the 20 percent in fact had a valid reason to deviate from the algorithm.

A few physicians, for example, told us their patients didn't have an isolated symptom of chest pain. They might have had an arrhythmia, which led the treatment down a different path. Those doctors used the algorithm to a certain point with each patient and then took liberties to make adjustments. When the team recognized they had the freedom to deviate, it proved that we weren't enforcing a dogmatic system across the board. We simply wanted to know the reason for each adjustment so we could use the information to continually make care for chest pain better.

We did, however, hold each team member accountable for three key measures or questions, not for the sake of grading them, but for the sake of refining the algorithm:

1. Did you use the stratification, the HEART score (History, EKG, Age, Risk factors, Troponin blood test) to determine the patient's level of risk for a serious heart problem? If not, why?
2. Disposition of the patient (home, observation, or in-patient)?
3. Did the patient come back within the next month, for any reason?

That's it. We found physicians and nurses put more meaningful thought into those three simple questions than they might when filling out dozens and dozens of data points, as they are not always sure what they are looking for. They hope to determine what they are looking for from analyzing the data points.

Another valuable takeaway from the Pilot Phase: It gives a glimpse at how well people will manage themselves when given the power and flexibility to focus on the patient. In a healthcare setting, their minds *want* to use all possible input synthetically. They know, almost instinctively, that consideration of every nuance is the best method. It's a natural desire that the systematic use of data has diluted. We've found that the synthetical approach inspires medical staffs to explore solutions to problems and feed them back into the cycle, which continues to turn and grow and improve. The methodology is, above all else, exactly what we claim it to be: doing whatever is best for the patient.

Phase 3: Implement

Ambassadors Out Front Expand the Bandwidth

We know the temptation. The Design and Pilot are the less flashy phases. You'll want to rush through them and get to the tangible phase: Implement. But don't give in to the desire to roll out a shiny new program as quickly and as dramatically as possible. A transformative method of care will wither if it's just "different." It has to be proven at the front lines. It has to involve everyone. And it has to be accepted before it's implemented.

Again, if you skip or hasten any step, the entire cycle will flame out as quickly as a Roman candle.

Auto designers have learned important lessons about patience. Take the viability of electric power. The first go-round with electric cars back in the early 1970s didn't go so well.

Developers rushed the cars out to the trade shows with wild hopes that the public would embrace them for the novelty, for the desire of being "first." The public pretty much saw those cars as hair dryers on four wheels. They fizzled and disappeared. There's been far more care and consideration in the latest iteration, with input from focus groups, dealers, and end users. Gradually, automakers have improved the battery technology, weight distribution, performance, and functionality. Instead of offering electric-only cars, they made adjustments to what are now gas-electric hybrid vehicles. It's doubtful these cars would be as popular as they are now had the design teams just said, "Here's the electric car we conceived in our heads. Hope you like it."

> "If anything goes bad, I did it. If anything goes semi-good, we did it. If anything goes really good, then *you* did it."
>
> —Coach Paul "Bear" Bryant

Frontline relationships are the driving forces in the bridge between acceptance and the Implement Phase. It isn't practical for two or three people to come down from an office and engage in meaningful conversations with thousands of doctors. A group of administrators will only appear to be issuing orders, even if it isn't their intent. Implementation is also ineffective when we rely on booklets or emails or webcasts—anything that's readable and deletable might be helpful but will certainly be forgotten. Your coalition needs to be the deliverer of the message to the front line. That's how you combine scale with power.

For us, we knew that one emergency medical group covers all ten of our emergency departments. So, we empowered them to educate, person to person, the core emergency personnel in those ten hospitals. Those team members then helped educate their colleagues on the front lines, driving the message wide and deep.

Similarly, in cardiology, some of our physicians would say in response to the implementation of the algorithm, "Oh yeah, I had that idea eight years ago."

We'd say, "Really? Someone should have been listening back then. It's a good thing you're a few steps ahead. In fact, we need you to help us implement this with the rest of your cardiology team."

We encouraged the doctors not only to share the methodology but also to *take credit for any successes from it*.

Paul "Bear" Bryant is a legendary college football coach and motivator. He had a humble manner about winning, which fostered more of it. He said, "If anything goes bad, *I* did it. If anything goes semi-good, *we* did it. If anything goes really good, then *you* did it."

Coach Bryant knew that when people share in the credit of success, it lights a fire. This is why we want everyone on our medical teams to participate in the Implement Phase. Each person can see the methodology at play. Each person has the freedom to adjust it and write down the reason for the adjustment. And each person feels responsible when it works.

Pretty quickly, we have a strong network of medical ambassadors working cohesively as active, living change agents.

Phase 4: Sustain

When "the Other" Kinds of Change Blow Through

You get to a point where everything starts to click. Physicians and nurses are using the algorithm as second nature. The influence of the coalition is contagious. Everyone is motivated, regaining a sense of purpose for patient-centric care.

And then . . . the nurse who believed in the methodology from the very start announces she's moving. The most respected physician on the team retires. They are two of your high-powered energy sources, and without them the momentum you've built is at risk of stopping. In a traditional model of change, you might be in trouble.

In a transformed model, you have nothing to worry about.

It's going to happen. Every year, there's a 20 percent turnover in nursing staff. A new group of attendings arrives in July, and there's a good chance they've been trained somewhere else in a different system. You want to keep good people, but if a few personnel changes undo whatever you've done, then the truth is, you never did reach the Sustain Phase. When you do get to this phase, the cycle will keep turning, no matter who is on the team.

We can't pinpoint exactly when we transitioned into this phase—and maybe that's the beauty of it. At some point people started saying about the algorithm, "This is the way we've *always* gone about treating patients here," even though it isn't. When a new nurse or physician arrives, the people on the front line take the initiative to show them the key measures. The new person will say, "Where did this come from?" And that's the opening for the frontline staff to explain how they were personally involved in the development of the design, the pilot, and the implementation.

> The very reason the pathway can be sustained through winds of change is that it is *not* etched in stone.

Whether they know it or not, they just happen to be living out the Sustain Phase. It's like muscle memory. It becomes embedded in the patient care.

Yet the very reason the pathway can be sustained through winds of change is that it is *not* etched in stone. It can be adjusted, with valid reasons. And because of that, the pathway is fluid enough to transcend generations, timelines, and standards . . . and always move forward.

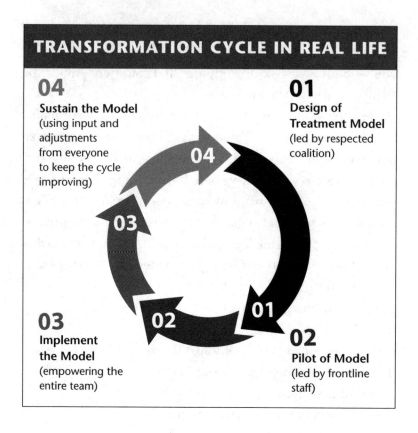

Fully Transformed

So, how do you know when you've run the four phases and have actually *transformed* a method of care? There is no objective test. The evidence is in what you see, touch, and hear.

We knew we'd transformed the way we treat chest pain when we received a phone call from a hospital on the other side of Florida. An attending who had recently moved there from our hospital was on the phone, saying, "Can you believe our emergency department here doesn't use the HEART score? They don't use the algorithm at all!" This person was appalled that they weren't following the pathway of care he'd learned at our hospital. He then said, "Can you send the algorithm to me? I want to show it to our team here."

That's when we realized the change the medical team had designed, piloted, and implemented was fully acculturated as the best way to care for chest-pain patients.

We've explored pathways for twenty-six different conditions. At this moment, we're actively moving eighteen of them through the phases on the spectrum. Some are fully transformed. But we've also learned from the other eight pathways that stalled during the early phases. In one, we didn't have a strong enough champion on the coalition. For another, the potential win didn't justify the energy necessary to make it happen. We identified permanent barriers that suggested it wasn't the right time for a particular pathway. But those projects are not failures. They didn't consume copious resources and time. In fact, we treat the notes from our early conversations like the excess screws and nuts you have left over when assembling furniture. Instead of throwing the dialogue away, we keep the input and the lessons in a little box. Then we use them as we start up another pathway, because they might be exactly what we need to tie solutions to certain problems.

There's one very important link in these phases: the simple act of gathering physicians together to participate in a meaningful mission. When they know their expertise is valued and that we have a shared purpose, the collaboration alone infuses strength into the pathway. Then the strength grows when they see for themselves: a flexible algorithm in writing, with their own signatures on it. The influence is exponential.

The power of the pathway, remember, starts on the front line and flexes out from there. It exists because the medical team is *em*powered. They become confident enough to use the methodology to treat a specific condition, and then extend it to other clinical problems. They believe it. They use it. They believe it again. They use it again. The cycle of transformation is in motion.

KEY POINTS FROM CHAPTER SEVEN

- **Empower the front line.** Giving doctors an opportunity to create a plan and then allowing them to use it is important. We encouraged the doctors who helped develop the methodology to not only share it but also to take credit for any successes from it.

- **The transformation timeline.** The design phase does not take nearly as much time as you might think. Our coalition agreed on a vision and algorithm and removed the barriers to implementing them in 4–5 weeks.

- **Deviations are okay.** Flexibility is another way to bring everyone on board for the ride and to rekindle the passion for appropriate personalized care. Deviations, even slight ones, provide valuable insight to improve the methodology.

- **Spreading the plan most effectively.** It's important to give credit for success to the people working directly with the patients. Bear Bryant recognized that when people share in the credit of success, it lights a fire.

- **A sign of transformation.** You know change is firmly embedded into the culture when staff believe you have always done it that way. And when physicians who have moved away want to share the algorithm with their new team.

REFLECTIONS

- At the end of chapter three, you identified an area of patient care where current protocols slow down diagnosis and treatment and/or create unnecessary costs. You also wrote down the names of people who would best merge synthetical thinking into that area of care (people who are knowledgeable, personable, and whom frontline workers respect).

- Invite those people to meet on the subject of creating and leading a transformative plan for patient care.

- Ask them to:
    - formulate a vision to improve that area of care.
    - agree on the components of an algorithm and to write down the algorithm.
    - dentify the barriers to change, and how they would remove those barriers.

- Have the coalition members sign the consensus-written algorithm. Give them ownership of it.

CHAPTER 8

Healthcare Beyond Recognition

Change Isn't "Transformation" Until It's Permanent

Two events at sunrise have mesmerized me since I (Danny) moved to Florida. On the Atlantic coast, I can watch the sun in all of its glory as it seems to slowly emerge from the ocean. It's a reminder of our awesome Creator, sending that fiery ball of life-giving light every 24 hours. The second event at sunrise isn't nearly as grand, but to me is still a spectacle. This event is the insects, their shapes and tints coming to life as the sun starts to dry the dew from the grass and leaves.

One insect that really catches my eye is the dragonfly. Those beautiful iridescent colors sparkle when the early sun shines on them. In those moments, it's hard to comprehend the previous life of the dragonfly. It is a story of complete transformation.

The dragonfly doesn't enter its existence as a dragonfly. It moves through stages—from unattractive egg to unattractive nymph before hatching as something altogether new and beautiful, the dragonfly. The nymph (or larvae) can take a few years to mature while living in water. When it finally sheds its skin . . . *wow*.

Here's the catch for the dragonfly. Once it's transformed from nymph to dragonfly, it cannot go back to its former self. The change is permanent. It has undergone *transformation*.

The word transformation is used a lot these days—and is often *mis*-used. All transformation is change. But not all change is transformation. The nymph changing to a dragonfly? That's transformation. And that's the kind of trajectory we need in healthcare, the type of change where there's no turning back, where no one even *wants* to turn back.

The Four "Musts" for Transformation

Transformation does not come as naturally for us as it does for the dragonfly. We need to *make* it happen. Change only becomes transformative when we're committed to implementing it into the living, breathing cycle of our daily work. One or two people can't do this. All attempts at permanent change fail if even a few people don't believe in it and participate. It's like leaving the top off the toothpaste and thinking, "Oh well, I'm going to use it again in a few hours anyway, and besides, someone else always seems to put the top back on."

That's why transformation in healthcare has to start at the macro level—not with the executives or the people who develop the ten-year vision. Everyone from the front line to the front office has to be a participant, embedding the change into the culture.

We identified four "musts" as our coalition developed methods of care for chest pain, syncope, and sepsis:

1. We must . . . empower the front line.
2. We must . . . hold them accountable with reasonable measures.

3. We must . . . embed the methodology into the workflow. It isn't a separate component. It can't be time-consuming. It isn't a list of items that "I'll try to get around to." If a team helps build it, then they'll be enthused to use it and willing to be held accountable for their own measures.
4. We must . . . transform our thinking to continually improve without end.
   People associate a goal with a finish line—a rapid-cycle improvement. With transformation, *there is no finish line.* Everyone is permanently growing and improving. It's one patient, one life at a time. Someone in another office can crunch the numbers. Our goal is to save lives.

Transformation #1: Chest Pain

Chest pain represents 10 percent of the adult medical issues in the emergency department. It's by far the highest number of unanticipated admissions to the hospital. Once our coalition came up with an algorithm to determine whether to release patients, admit them, or hold them for further observation, the question was, "How do we embed the algorithm into the workflow?"

The embedding would be the difference between a) completely transforming our care for chest pain or b) making a change—a rapid-cycle improvement—knowing it may eventually revert back.

In medical school and in nurse training, you learn acronyms to regurgitate for exams. The acronyms and their application become second nature only if you use them in real-life situations every day. Remember, a physician makes hundreds of decisions during the normal working day, so an acronym that's useful every now and then will be buried under a pile of information.

One well-known acronym for chest pain is the HEART score: History, EKG, Age, Risk factors for heart disease, and the Troponin blood test. Useful as it is, the HEART score is one of those methods that's often lost in a sea of daily decision making. So, our coalition decided to embed the HEART score into something we're always tied to, the electronic medical record. You can't miss information on the EMR screen—it is constantly in front of us.

After we integrated the HEART score into the EMR, it went from a five-step method that physicians would randomly use from time to time . . . to a part of our culture. In every case of chest pain, the EMR now shows us the EKG recorded in the system, the age in the permanent record, the risk factors we know and have validated, and the results of the blood test. That's the objective data, or the EART. And it leads each physician to examine the H—history—to complete the score. This is the all-important patient-doctor relationship.

"How severe is the pain and where?"

"Does it radiate?"

"What were you doing when this happened?"

As a physician or nurse, you never know what kind of valuable information you might glean unless you engage the patient in conversation. You can also read the body language and other nonverbal cues. The data in EART are helpful, but the changeover really comes when it's wrapped into the H.

This process is not difficult. It isn't as complex as artificial intelligence or as expensive as rolling more technology into the room. You're using:

- *Synthetical thinking*: The blending of objective information, subjective information, and expertise.
- *An algorithm*: This is the patient-specific HEART score. And it only takes a matter of minutes for everyone to learn.

Of all things, the prompt in the EMR has allowed us to embed the methodology—the change—into the culture. Transformation is underway in the way we treat chest pain, and there's no reason to go back.

ACTION LIST FOR CHEST PAIN METHODOLOGY

- ☐ Embed the HEART score into the EMR: History, EKG, Age, Risk Factors, Troponin (blood test).
- ☐ Emphasize the physician-patient conversation for History.
- ☐ Embed button for "Discharge" in EMR as part of the workflow.
- ☐ Schedule a follow-up with the patient within 72 hours.

Transformation #2: Syncope

The second high-risk, high-volume condition we see in the emergency departments is syncope. Syncope is when a person loses consciousness and postural tone. One moment they're standing in the kitchen and the next moment they're lying on the floor, and they don't know how they got there. Now they're in the hospital.

Our coalition knew how well the HEART score worked for chest pain once they integrated it into the EMR. The HEAD score works in a similar way for conditions that occur above the neck. It's the History, EKG, Age, and Diagnostic testing (the diagnostic might be the blood level of the hemoglobin or the hematocrit or the blood sugar value).

For our medical teams, the HEAD score is an aggregate of three scoring systems rolled into one comprehensive yet simple pathway for syncope decisions. We want a reassurance that "we aren't missing anything with this patient." So each letter in the HEAD simplifies a larger group of twenty-seven parameters. How we arrived at those twenty-seven parameters is as creative as it is logical.

In medical school you take a test to recognize a scoring system in cases of syncope to determine whether to keep the patient or discharge them. However, there are about six different scoring systems. The three most familiar systems are the Rose Risk Score, the San Francisco Syncope Rules, and OESIL Risk Score. In each of these three systems, you look at nine parameters. So the team said, "Let's aggregate all the parameters. If a patient is positive in any of those twenty-seven areas, it's a red flag. Conversely, if the patient shows zero of the twenty-seven signs, then we can confidently discharge and have them follow up with a doctor within 72 hours to determine the cause of the syncopal episode."

We've learned two significant lessons from the coalition's work on syncope—one lesson about innovation and the other about discharging patients.

The innovation from syncope is the idea to use three widely accepted methods and, instead of choosing one, combining them *into* one. We haven't lost a sensitive point in any of the methods, yet we aren't losing valuable time either. Rather than running the tests in a long series where results from one test necessitate another test and the results from that test require another test, we run all three tests parallel with each other. Think of a pregnancy test. A woman says, "Honey, I think I might be pregnant." So you go to the drugstore, buy three different brands of pregnancy tests, and run samples on all three at the same time. If even one is positive, well, the woman isn't one-third pregnant. It's all or nothing. She knows it's time to see her OB-GYN. In the same way, our methodology for syncope doesn't add time or resources, and yet medical personnel can be confident they haven't missed anything.

The discharge is another dramatic change we made. Our coalition realized the process of discharging a patient had become a huge barrier for physicians, specifically the follow-up appointment. Logically, discharging should be easier than moving a patient around the hospital for additional observation, but it doesn't work so easily. The typical electronic medical record doesn't include a prompt for discharging and scheduling a visit within 72 hours, say, the same way you'd push "checkout" when ordering a product online. The physician will say, "Make sure you see someone within a week or so," which is like giving someone a bus pass and hoping they'll use it someday. Then there's the extraneous process of filling out forms and sending the patient to another office on a different floor. For physicians and nurses, sometimes it's more efficient to hold the patient in the hospital as an inpatient and exhaust all the steps in the evaluation—even if they aren't necessary—rather than discharge the patient. It costs time and resources.

So we integrated a "magic button" on the EMR. When the provider pushes the button, the screen goes to an order for the care coordination center to set up a follow-up appointment within 72 hours. With this, the patient can go home faster with a simple plan in hand. He or she knows without a doubt their needs have been met. They haven't spent thousands of dollars on tests. The medical team is confident in the discharge because we've gone

> With transformation, there is no finish line. Everyone is permanently growing and improving.

through twenty-seven points of potential concern and we have a follow-up appointment scheduled just to be extra sure.

We're treating each patient with more personalized care. Money is saved. Everyone participates. The HEAD score is now embedded in the culture. Patients with syncope are in good hands. What's not to like?

ACTION LIST FOR SYNCOPE METHODOLOGY
- ☐ Look at 27 parameters involving history, observation, and feedback.
- ☐ If the patient has 0 signs out of 27 possibilities, discharge.
- ☐ Embed button for "Discharge" in EMR as part of the workflow.
- ☐ Schedule a follow-up with the patient within 72 hours.

Transformation #3: Sepsis

The most dangerous illness in healthcare environments worldwide is sepsis—an infection that can overtake the vital organs. It's by far the number-one cause of in-hospital deaths. The only way to stop sepsis is to discover it early, almost before the patient even realizes he or she is sick.

There are several tests we've used for sepsis over the years, but none could definitively tell us, "Yes, this is a septic problem. We need all hands on deck." We have a sepsis alert, which is triggered when there are changes in heart rate, degree of consciousness, or blood sugar levels. The alert says *conditions are right for a potential sepsis problem,* but it isn't a sure thing. It's like a weather alert for a tornado watch: nothing has been sighted yet, but the signs are here for the slightest possibility of a tornado. The sepsis alert is extremely iffy, and if we jump to heavy antibiotics prematurely, we could cause more harm than good.

One test really got our attention though: the NEWS2 score used primarily in the UK. The full acronym (National Early Warning System) sounds as if it were borrowed from the weather forecasters. The Royal College of Physicians developed NEWS2 in the early 2000s, and shortly after that the UK's National Health Service (NHS) adopted it. In order for the NHS to adopt it, it is required to go through NICE—National Institute for Clinical Excellence—an English governmental agency that brings together the best of *clinicians* to create the algorithms that then drive the entire NHS. Whereas traditional tests for sepsis only tell us "conditions are right" (akin to the tornado watch), the NEWS2 score takes us to the next level, the tornado warning or sepsis warning. It tells us, "An infection has been spotted and it's headed in your direction."

The NEWS2 score takes into account the patient's vital signs and level of consciousness to create a quantifiable single-digit score. Everyone on the team can read the results and easily communicate them by figuratively pulling an alarm. Like the tornado warning, the score tells us, "Sepsis has actually been spotted in this patient. Everyone, pay attention. You need to start treatment *now*."

As we went through the previous protocols for sepsis, we noted that ordering the treatment took valuable time. The order itself doesn't do any good. Waiting sure doesn't help. The only action that helps in a sepsis case is to actually pour the fluids and get the antibiotics into the patient. The body needs those antibiotics to neutralize and kill the microbes causing the infection. We call this a Sepsis Power Plan. It's an organized way for the physician to be assured, "Yes, I'm doing the six things needed to take care of this patient with sepsis." At the same time, it also sends the Power Plan to everyone who's involved in caring for the patient currently and who will be caring for the patient later, whether it's in the ICU or non-ICU.

For consistency, we use the same NEWS2 scoring to determine when the patient is improving. This is important because so often with illness we know when someone is sick, but we don't always take quick measures when they're getting better. It's important to change the medications and move the patient closer to being released home, where they can return to full health without the threat of a repeat infection.

The whole system (the NEWS2 score, the staff-wide notification, the Sepsis Power Plan) is easy and convenient to follow. For the patient, it is literally lifesaving. And because it's similar to the HEART score and HEAD score that we've already embedded, we can easily implement the NEWS2 score into our culture. Everyone participates. It's with us permanently.

> **ACTION LIST FOR SEPSIS METHODOLOGY**
> - ☐ Use the NEWS2 (National Early Warning System) single-digit score derived from patient's vital signs and level of consciousness, among other factors.
> - ☐ Determine if an infection has been spotted.
> - ☐ Use Sepsis Power Plan by delivering fluids into the body so the antibiotics go to work—don't wait.

How Do You Know the Change Is Permanent?

When a nymph changes into a dragonfly, there's no mistaking it. The insect takes on a whole different look. The change in how we practice healthcare might not be as obvious at a glance as the emergence of a dragonfly. But take a step closer.

When you observe a team on the front line using the HEART score without hesitation, when you hear them say, "I know what's causing the chest pain because I've used the HEART score," you know the care is different.

When a patient passes out, you don't hear, "Hmm. I wonder what caused that." Instead, you see the medical team go right to the HEAD score for syncope.

When a sick patient at the onset of sepsis is receiving fluids because the team has said, "The NEWS2 score told us to pull the alarm and start the Sepsis Power Plan," you can be sure the culture of healthcare in that area has changed for good.

Lives are being saved. Medical teams are confident about their work and enthused about the outcomes. Patients are going home faster, happier, and healthier. You're witnessing an incredible, permanent change. This is transformation. We are never going back.

KEY POINTS FROM CHAPTER EIGHT

- **The four transformation *musts*.** We identified four *musts* as our coalition developed methods of care for chest pain, syncope, and sepsis: empowering the front line, holding them accountable with reasonable measures, embedding a methodology in the workflow, and transforming the "finish line" mindset.

- **The EMR as our ally.** We embedded the 5-step HEART score into the EMR for chest-pain patients to help integrate it into our workflow and culture.

- **A transformed plan for syncope.** We synthesized three scoring systems into one, called the HEAD score, and created a "magic button" on the EMR. It's faster, more accurate, and less costly.

- **A transformed plan for sepsis.** We adopted the NEWS2 scoring system, developed a Sepsis Power Plan, and ensured the plan was communicated to all necessary staff. This easy-to-use early warning system saves thousands of lives.

- **No turning back.** When our work is transformed by effective strategies created by the front line, there's no desire to return to old ways.

REFLECTIONS

- Ask the coalition to communicate its concise vision for patient care to frontline staff.

- Ask them to share the new methodology for that area of care to frontline staff.

- Empower leaders on the front line to implement the algorithm.

- Embed into the workflow a way for everyone to track each time the algorithm is used or not used, plus a reason each time the algorithm is not used.

- The coalition and frontline leaders remind everyone there are no specific goals or finish lines at this point. The algorithm will constantly be adjusted based on feedback and synthetical thinking.

CHAPTER 9

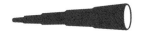

Saving Thousands of Lives & Millions of Dollars

This Is Transformation You Can Count

From an insider's perspective, I've (Danny) noticed an interesting correlation between healthcare and law enforcement. Specifically, it's the way we use resources when a problem arises—real or not. One incident from my law enforcement days epitomizes this.

On this particular morning, my investigative team was on patrol when an urgent call came over the radio. The call was vague but frantic. The dispatcher said, "We've got a major problem. I have a woman on the phone screaming. Everyone needs to mobilize toward the location."

So all of these units started rolling into this neighborhood—SWAT teams, undercover cars, vans, you name it. Blues and twos, as we termed it, with our lights and sirens screaming in from every direction, some skidding sideways. At this point we only know a female was in distress. She was still screaming. Dozens of us put on firearms and vests before using brute force to crash down the garden gate and run toward the door. When I say we hit the door, I mean we *hit the door*—so hard it literally came off its hinges. Once in the house, we fanned out to contain the danger at hand. As I was barking out orders, I spotted the woman at the top of the stairs; she was still frantic about something.

"What's the issue?" I asked.

She pointed at the base of the stairway. "There! There!" she shouted.

I looked around and finally found, not far from my feet, a frog. All I could do was collect myself, settle the adrenaline, and casually call everyone off. We had mobilized everything in our arsenal—officers, vehicles, weapons, communications systems—because a woman needed to be rescued from a frog that was hanging out at the bottom of her stairs. We were thankful the woman and frog would be fine. That said, there's no telling how much money we invested into this emergency. It's very possible we endangered the well-being of other citizens who truly did need our help at this moment. Unfortunately, we poured all our resources into this frog call.

We do the same kind of thing in healthcare. When a perceived threat goes off, the best move would be to take a breath, ask questions, and use subjective information to make a proper decision. That's synthetical thinking in a nutshell. But instead, "modern healthcare" tells us we need to surround the situation with physicians, nurses, time, resources, and endless technology. Oftentimes, it's like the frog—the threat amounts to something minor. Yet the costs are heavy.

Who Pays for All of This?

Today, for the first time in history, individuals pay more of the healthcare dollar than insurance companies and government programs. The numbers are staggering when you add up all the copays, premiums, deductibles, and out-of-pocket expenses. A big part of the problem is that on a day-to-day basis we default to worst-case possibilities. It might sound like the right thing to do, in theory. But it isn't, especially when we usher patients through costly diagnostics and Star Trekkie tests, even when they aren't necessary. When we overadmit patients, the dollar figures escalate. And while these resources are heaped on a patient who might or might not need them, another patient who *does* need heightened care could be in peril while waiting for those resources to be freed up.

Here is the other version of our cartoon with the patient sitting on an exam table with an arrow through his head. In this version, the doctor looks up from his electronic medical record, locks his eyes on the arrow, and finally says, "I think I know what the problem is . . . but I'm going to order some tests just to be sure."

A traditional thought process is common between hospitals and hospitality: heads in beds. Just admit the patients. We can work out the issue once they're in a room. It's like taking your car to the dealership and saying, "The steering feels a little off. I'm pretty sure my tires need to be rotated." But instead of listening to you and rotating the tires, they decide to hold the car for two days while they also change the gaskets and overhaul the transmission.

This isn't treating the patient, or the owner of the vehicle, as your first, second, or third priority. It might seem caring to say, "Let's throw everything we've got at this." But the ramifications to the patient are enormous. We're adding to their angst the weight of costs for tests and a room. The hospital also has to pay for staffing and space. Then there's the risk of hospital-acquired conditions (C. diff and MRSA) whenever we place patients who might not be sick near people who are acutely sick.

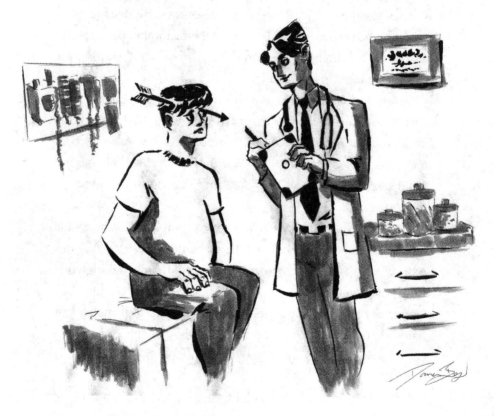

"I think I know what the problem is . . .
but I'm going to order some tests just to be sure."

© MMXXI AdventHealth Press. Used by permission.

These stresses—financial, spatial, and medical—fall on the patient *and* on our ability to deliver the best healthcare. So the environment of today's healthcare system is the perfect test bed for a transformative methodology. While that sounds like an academic term, in practice it's the opposite. Anyone can use this methodology to relieve our most pressing burdens without directives from some ivory tower. We've done it ourselves, starting with one patient, then a few more.

The results? In only a few years and in a handful of hospitals, we've saved millions of dollars and thousands of lives—literally.

The Ideal Test Bed

The highest patient volume in our hospitals comes from people experiencing chest pain. In a sense, it's at the top of our funnel. Within our healthcare system, under one hospital license in a city of three million people, more than 4,000 patients a month present to the eight emergency departments with chest pain. As soon as we begin to move those patients through the funnel, we also begin to build up the stresses of cost, resources, and risk.

Typically, a patient comes into the ED and says, "I'm having chest pain." They're taken into a space for testing. First, it's an EKG. Then there are a variety of blood tests (but not the basic troponin test we use on the algorithm). The team might order an ultrasound. Perhaps a CAT scan. They'll do a transesophageal echocardiogram. Oh, and let's go ahead and give this patient a stress test—either the one where they can just lie in the bed and receive an injection of a medication or where they actually get up and run around the bed a few times and are evaluated.

From there, the decision is almost always on the ultraconservative side. "Well, chances are one in 100 this is necessary, but we're going to err on the side of admitting the patient to the hospital." And there you go. The car in need of a tire rotation is on the lift for a two-day stay.

We do all of this because "modern healthcare" warns us that you don't want to risk missing something and having the patient die or continue to suffer from an undetected serious medical problem. So, we admit them even when the symptoms don't warrant it. The physician might know this is a temporary discomfort *not* related to a heart attack or life-threatening heart disease. But analytical thinking in the current system says to test, test, test, and admit.

This is why we started with a blank slate at the top of the funnel—the moment when the patient enters the ED with chest pain. We said, "Forget the current protocols for now. As experienced physicians who are passionate about helping people, what should we do as soon as *that* patient comes through *that* door?" Take every bit of information into account—personal, practical, historical, relational—and think through a solution synthetically.

It took very little time before we agreed the HEART score would be a much-needed dramatic change. The physicians wanted a stratification tool to shift their approach from "let's test and admit" to "trust the algorithm and deliver the best care possible." That means identify each patient as high, medium, and low risk, and *then* decide whether to send them for tests or to send them home.

To be clear, we'll still send patients who obviously need their arteries opened up directly to the cath lab. They'll always be provided the immediate lifesaving help they need. The HEART score applies to the patients in the "uncertain" segment who make up the majority of chest-pain presentations to the ED. With that, we knew we could potentially save time and resources. We just weren't sure how much we'd save . . . or how many lives.

The "Before"

We started with those 4,000 patients per month with chest pain. In the baseline years, before we piloted and implemented our methodology, the segmentation looked like this:

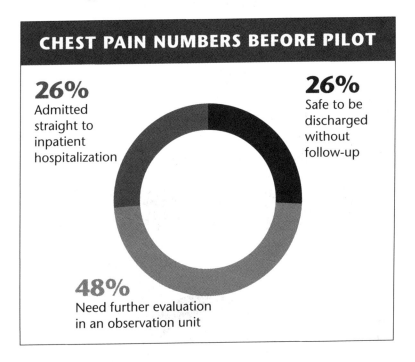

We found that the 26 percent of patients who had been cleared for discharge spent several hours in the emergency department with significant variation in how they'd been evaluated and treated. Few followed up after being discharged.

The 48 percent who went to the observation unit would spend about a day and a half there being tested. The vast majority of them were not experiencing a heart attack.

Then, the 26 percent of chest-pain patients who were admitted—whether they had something go wrong or not—spent three and a half to four days in the inpatient unit. You often spend a day settling into the hospital, a day getting cardiology consultation, and a day being tested. Some would also go to the cath lab for a diagnostic catheterization of the arteries. A few would go into surgery or some form of intervention, like a stent or balloon angioplasty.

The "After"

Today, with the algorithm implemented and key measures being used to sustain it, we see a dramatically different story. An idea from the renegades in the corner has grown through synthetical thinking to bear enormous results. Honestly, we did not anticipate these in the beginning:

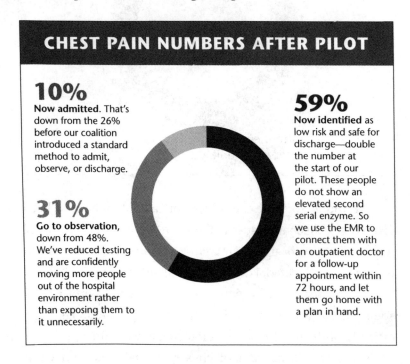

CHEST PAIN NUMBERS AFTER PILOT

10%
Now admitted. That's down from the 26% before our coalition introduced a standard method to admit, observe, or discharge.

31%
Go to observation, down from 48%. We've reduced testing and are confidently moving more people out of the hospital environment rather than exposing them to it unnecessarily.

59%
Now identified as low risk and safe for discharge—double the number at the start of our pilot. These people do not show an elevated second serial enzyme. So we use the EMR to connect them with an outpatient doctor for a follow-up appointment within 72 hours, and let them go home with a plan in hand.

By sheer numbers, that's 4,000 patients a month with chest pain. Today we have 1,000 fewer patients staying in the hospital. Of those, 700 do not need to be admitted for inpatient care. The differential of the 3.5-day stay (for admission) and the 1.5-day stay (for observation) has changed our daily census by about 100 patients.

The traditional healthcare administrators and finance officers will look at these numbers and start to feel chest pain themselves. *Where are the heads in beds?*

The methodology doesn't follow a business model. It follows what's best for the patient, which turns out to be best for *everyone*. Low-risk patients are not taking up 100 beds on any given day. We followed all those patients who had been released within the pilot for thirty days and found no instance of a major adverse cardiac event (MACE). Zero. Releasing them is the best decision.

Think about it. Those 100 beds are open instead for patients who are fighting for their lives. They might be experiencing an organ failure. They might need lifesaving transplants. Or they're sepsis patients who need higher-level care in an intensive care unit or progressive care unit or med-surgical unit. We should always have beds available for them.

All of this happens to be best for the hospital, too. Whereas before we couldn't take severely ill patients from out of system because the chest-pain patients were in the beds waiting for more tests, we can now accept these people and give them proper care. The "No Vacancy" sign now says, "Come. Let our well-trained team make you better in your time of great need."

Everyone wins, starting with the patient.

Making Dollars from Sense

The cost comparisons from before and after the methodology are startling as well:

DIRECT COST COMPARISONS FOR CHEST PAIN PATIENTS
Admitting a Patient
$3,500 average (labor, supplies, doctors' fees)
Holding a Patient for Observation
$1,500 (labor, supplies, tests)
Evaluating and Releasing a Patient
$500 (with follow-up appointment confirmed)

From there, the direct-cost analysis is pretty simple. Take just one year and 1,000 fewer patients held per month—700 are admissions and 300 are observations. Multiply those by the cost savings of moving them from inpatient to outpatient. The direct cost in our healthcare system alone is $32 million of opportunity each year.

We have identified the opportunity to save tens of millions of dollars, just for doing what's best for the patient.

The patient saves money. The hospital saves money. Communities have more money to spend on important projects. Employers who send patients to healthcare systems don't have to raise the prices of their goods and services. And insurance companies don't have to raise premiums. Huge burdens are lifted. And it's logical to think that with less financial stress we should see healthier people in mind, body, and spirit.

Of course, the $32 million will only have that kind of widespread impact if healthcare providers adjust staffing ratios and reallocate expertise to where it needs to go. But that's another advantage in the big picture. People don't lose jobs. Their skills are instead linked to the type of care that's needed most. The sense of purpose returns.

We could go on and on with the benefits. In short, the changes foster good stewardship of our time, talents, and treasures.

Now let's pull back from the emergency department and take a wider-angle view of capital investments. If chest-pain patients still occupied 100 additional beds, the traditional model would entice us to build a new tower with 100 rooms. It looks nice. It becomes the talk of the town. Perhaps there's some economic value to the community. But there's also a significant cost. A hospital room for a patient being treated for chest pain costs about a million dollars. That's a $100 million project just to keep the 100 patients who didn't need to be admitted. Wouldn't it be better to reallocate the money to doing something else for real patient needs? Maybe it could be invested into community needs, or the intensive care units could be redesigned so patients can recover more fully at extended outpatient rehab and care facilities. Now *that* would be an extension of our ministry.

Healing from Hospitality

You hear four words said repeatedly in hospitals: "You need to rest." It's true. Without rest, the body will have a hard time recovering from illness and regaining strength. Some would argue rest is the most important factor in whole-person health. Just look at the onset of sepsis. The body needs energy to fight the infection.

But the reality is, we make it impossible for the patients to rest. We wake them up to take tests or to ask them if they were sleeping okay and we allow outside noise to filter into the rooms. The environment isn't conducive to complete rest. We need to soften the environment (and, by the way, noise is another good reason to discharge patients who might not even need inpatient care).

I (Danny) often imagine how much better a hospital environment would be if it were to align with what you find on the Appalachian Trail. The peacefulness, or soft noise, is one reason I'm such an avid hiker. There's a gentle rhythm in the forest and at the beach that's wholistically better than the hard noise in the city. So what if we were to take some of our savings from unnecessary admissions and invest it into a healing environment?

> In only a few years and in a handful of hospitals, we've saved millions of dollars and thousands of lives—literally.

We've seen this at a few healthcare facilities. There are hospitals in the US and abroad that have successfully worked with lawmakers to restrict noise from outside sources (cars, trains, nearby public venues). But when it comes to empathy for patient rest, Celebration Health in Central Florida has made real, meaningful investments. The main lobby and corridors are designed to remind patients of being in a Mediterranean-inspired hotel. Walk into the imaging department and you feel like you've gone to the beach. On the walls are ocean murals. Through the speakers are the sounds of seabirds. Changing rooms have been converted to beach cabanas. Patients wear flip-flops, island-style shirts, and baggy shorts rather than hospital gowns. A sense of peace replaces a sense of fear. The environment is so restful that the cancellation rate for imaging tests has dropped significantly, and patients who are admitted find themselves in rooms that are more resort-ish than hospital-ish. They have effectively embraced the long-lost healthcare principle of *hospitality*. Patients actually feel at rest.

Now consider what we all know: that rest coincides with health and healing. Rest can even stave off an avoidable worst-case scenario, like sepsis.

More Lives Saved

Our methodology for sepsis again stems from a common-sense synthetical mindset at the front line. How? By treating patients early and preventing long hospital stays. Before we introduced our coalition's algorithm, the mortality rate for sepsis in our hospital was around 22 percent, slightly better than the national average. After taking a wholistic approach and introducing NEWS2 and the Sepsis Power Plan, we reduced the mortality rate to 8 percent in the pilot.

How does a drop from 22 percent to 8 percent translate into saving lives? It represents 1,500 additional lives in two years. That's 1,500 patients who have walked out of the hospital rather than never making it. The value of 1,500 people to their families, friends, and contribution to society is immeasurable.

While the results are easy to add up on a spreadsheet, they're hard to fully comprehend in terms of importance to the greater good. Keep in mind, we've seen these dramatic outcomes in only a few years and in a few hospitals. Chest pain and sepsis are just two of the important conditions we care for—there are others to address. But we've taken the first long steps to prove we can save millions of dollars and thousands of lives at the grassroots level, which tells us this is just the beginning of transformation.

KEY POINTS FROM CHAPTER NINE

- **Financial burdens.** Individuals now pay more of the healthcare dollar than insurance companies and government programs, including the unnecessary costs.

- **The cost of reactionary healthcare.** Oftentimes we default to a worst-case possibility and use unnecessary and costly diagnostic tools, creating needless expense for the patient. Resources need to be spared for everyone's good.

- **Saving $32 million.** The strategy and the result of our chest-pain algorithm at one hospital proved its effectiveness by saving the hospital $32 million every year.

- **And another $100 million.** The simple changes we implemented for chest pain translate to capital savings of $100 million by reducing heads in beds, making room for patients that urgently need to be admitted.

- **Saving 1,500 lives.** The Sepsis Power Plan reduced one hospital's mortality rate by nearly two-thirds, saving 1,500 lives in just the pilot project.

- **The hospital environment.** We can and should invest in rest and a wholistic healing environment to improve patient outcomes.

- **Think bigger.** We've saved millions of dollars and thousands of lives from plans for chest pain and sepsis. What's stopping all of us from doing more?

REFLECTIONS

- Write out how your coalition's new plan for care will save resources for the patient's benefit.

- Write out how your coalition's new plan for care will save resources for the hospital's benefit.

- Write out how your coalition's new plan for care will save lives and promote health and healing.

CHAPTER 10

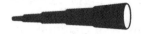

Moonshot Innovations

Rewards from Exploring the Frontier of Healthcare

In May of 1961, President John F. Kennedy told the world that the United States would do the unthinkable: We would send a man to the moon, land him on the untouched distant sphere, and bring him back safely to earth. We would accomplish this by the end of the decade. The mission he outlined generated a fair amount of skepticism, but mostly it inspired Americans everywhere to reimagine what might be possible. For the remainder of the 1960s, and for decades to follow, people would feel free to share bold ideas that previously had been buried under status quos and fears of ridicule.

In his speech about a moonshot, the president also mentioned possible outgrowths from the space exploration program. The ingenuity it took to build a spaceship and launch it to a gravity-deprived dot in the sky would spawn weather satellites and worldwide communications systems. Turns out, the possibilities he laid out were the basic seeds of innovation. The space program gave us technology for robotics, smoke detectors, artificial limbs, wireless connections, memory foam, satellite TV, smartphones, and advancements that to this day are still in the works.

Those are tangible benefits we can use today. But the nontangible benefits during the early space program were even more transformational. The space mission unified the American people from diverse backgrounds—not only the ones calculating the math for the space launch, but all across the country. Hundreds of thousands of Americans worked directly or indirectly on the project, and millions more paid close attention to its progress, giving rise to a shared purpose that everyone could rally around.

On the day of the launch, July 16, 1969, at Kennedy Space Center in Florida, politicians, celebrities, sports figures, well-known businesspeople, and everyday citizens gathered to watch history. The lead-up to launch erased divisions of race, gender, and political party. In fact, leaders of the Southern Christian Leadership Conference (SCLC) traveled to the Space Coast intending to protest the money being spent on the moon mission. But after watching the launch firsthand, the head of the SCLC, Dr. Ralph Abernathy, said, "I was one of the proudest Americans as I stood on this spot."

Later, former President Lyndon Johnson said, "It seemed as if the half million people who worked on the program were there lifting the Apollo 11."

The mission reminded us of an innate desire, which has been present throughout creation, to be innovators, to be frontiersmen. First, it was crossing the oceans to come to uncharted land. Then, it was the march west from the Eastern Seaboard, crossing through rugged landscape and moving from sea to shining sea. Once conquered, the frontiers—and the fear of the unknown—changed for good.

President Kennedy had resurrected that same American spirit around space exploration.

It is not overly dramatic to equate the commitment around the Apollo 11 mission to what we're up against today in healthcare. It seems like a world away. It's urgent. Every American needs it. And it's possible to make it happen if we all believe in the mission and the possibilities. There are no "maybes." It is a must.

Well, it so happens that a few months before the president's proclamation about the space program, a 13-year-old boy traveled with his father from Takoma Park, Maryland, to attend the presidential inauguration, a bitter cold day in January of 1961. On that day, President Kennedy famously said, "Ask not what your country can do for you, ask what you can do for your country."

Perhaps inspired by both speeches, that boy grew up to be the chief clinical officer for AdventHealth—David Moorhead. If you remember, Dr. Moorhead is the one who encouraged our small team with his own challenge: "We have our own moonshot opportunity in healthcare. And now you have the freedom to create change."

The Barriers between Us and Quality Patient Care

Healthcare needs to be different—the way we deliver it, the way we charge for it, and the way Americans perceive and trust it. But until Dr. Moorhead expressly gave us the freedom to explore, we didn't necessarily believe meaningful change could be on the near horizon. Had we known it was out there, we certainly weren't sure how we'd get there. Even as we moved forward with ideas to save lives and money, none of us realized the moonshot innovations that were about to come along for the ride.

We can link our trepidation to steadfast protocols in healthcare. They create barriers, some of them palpable and many of them woven into the system. We had to specifically identify those barriers and write them down, just as the Apollo 11 engineers had to do when mathematically figuring out how to safely send a manned aircraft nearly 240,000 miles from Earth. For us, it's sometimes the little hindrances that cost so much money and put lives at risk, like not having proper medication near the emergency department or in the imaging department. Over time, we tend to just "live with the inconvenience" because it's too frustrating to try to change a longstanding protocol. When we allow those barriers to stand, it means patient care isn't as safe, effective, timely or *important* as it should be.

However, there's an advantage to facing barriers. They become reasons for innovations.

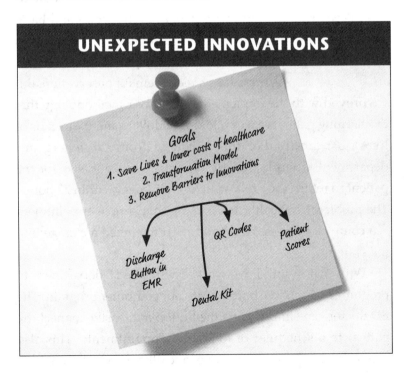

The Discharge Button

The hospital where we work emphasizes whole-person health. The body, mind, and spirit are all interconnected, so rather than compartmentalize our care, we attempt to treat it all. That means healthcare the way we define it doesn't start when you enter the hospital and end when you leave. Good health is continuous. We want to know how you're doing after you've come for treatment, whatever it might be. Releasing people to go home and following up should be the easy part. But it is far from true.

> There's an advantage to facing barriers. They become reasons for innovation.

Most hospitals in America make sending a patient home and seeing another doctor three days later as difficult as sending a person to the moon and back. The pathway in the system is set up to make it simple for physicians to admit patients or keep them for observation. But we proved with the implementation of our methodology that discharging patients saves millions of dollars and thousands of lives, just locally. For the discharge from the emergency department to work, though, we had to make it easy for the patient to return for a follow-up appointment within 72 hours. The problem? In healthcare, making that simple appointment is a complex process. We would need to embed a change into the system.

With that in mind, we worked with the IT department to program a "discharge button" into our computer program. The ED doctor can simply press the button and easily connect the patient to a scheduler of follow-up appointments. This also prompts the patient to leave a callback number, which previously would have been buried among a pile of paperwork.

Now, a simple button on a touchscreen breaks down a once-ominous barrier. Instead of defaulting to admission or a series of unnecessary tests, our physicians and nurses can be confident using the discharge prompt, knowing a medical specialist will be seeing the patient within three days. It's a seamless way to ensure the patient is healthy and to continue our relationship with the patient after he or she has gone home.

The Dental Kit

Toothache is a condition we see frequently in emergency departments. If a person feels the need to come in because of a toothache, you know the pain must be agonizing. A severe toothache can be a periodontal abscess, a localized infection with pus and significant swelling. The treatment is drainage of the infection and repair of the tooth by a dentist. This makes it painful for our ED team to say, "I'm sorry. There's nothing we can do. You'll need to see your dentist."

That's how the system works. We can't help you in your time of pain other than managing the symptoms with narcotics; we can't address the cause.

It was strange for me (Danny) to come to the US and find out the eyes and teeth are not considered part of the body in the American healthcare system—whomever came up with that idea was obviously thinking analytically and not synthetically. The insurances for vision and dental are separate, so people can come in with excruciating dental pain . . . and we can't do anything for them. It's incredibly frustrating. The only option other than sending the ailing patient away is for the doctor to admit them into the hospital. It's a costly alternative just for the sake of giving the patient some antibiotics until they can go to a dental specialist.

Our doctors told us, "We're supposed to help these people, not send them away." The way insurance separates the teeth from the rest of the body is the barrier in the way. So we implemented a dental kit. The emergency department physicians can now provide antibiotics and pain control right away. They don't simply write a prescription for the patient to go out and fill; the medical team is authorized to physically give the patient the medication so the healing process can start immediately and set the patient up for success with an appointment to a dentist.

Think of it as a starter kit to extend healthcare beyond the walls of the hospital, all the way to the dentist's office. The medicine holds the infection in check until an oral specialist can efficiently drill into the tooth or perform surgery. Relief comes from treatment and pain medication. Antibiotics may keep the abscess at bay until definitive treatment.

The patient gains the benefit of relief. The dentist gains the benefit of performing a procedure on a tooth less infected. The hospital gains the benefit of providing much-needed care without a costly stay. What started as a commitment to connect a few dots for the good of a patient with oral pain morphed into a dental kit you can touch. What were our prerequisites to make it happen? Common sense and a willingness to create change.

It isn't rocket science.

The QR Codes

In the early 2000s, fishermen in Jamaica started noticing fewer fish and dirtier water along the island's south coast. A group of local people concerned about the ocean habitat tried to convince the fishermen to do their fishing in deeper water, away from the reef system. The reef had been overfished to a point where there were no fish to keep it clean and healthy. Without a healthy reef, there would be no fish. However, the fishermen were from families who had made their livings from the reef for generations, so they dug in their heels and resisted. Their reliance on a convenient method became the biggest barrier to badly needed change.

The local group took a different approach. Rather than continually debating with the fishermen, they took them on field trips and showed them how reefs had been restored in other regions. The fishermen saw the abundance and size of fish in those places, and they became advocates for protecting the reef on their side of the island. More important, these long-time fishermen helped launch a foundation to educate people in their own communities about the value of protecting the reef. The local group successfully turned a huge barrier (the fishermen) into a solution to the problem.

> What were our prerequisites to make it happen? Common sense and a willingness to create change.

In healthcare (and in this book) we've identified the tablet or smartphone that a physician carries as a barrier in the physician-patient relationship (remember the doctor who didn't notice the arrow sticking through the guy's head?). We would never suggest eliminating computer screens. But we do know they can get in the way of a wholistic diagnosis at times.

So what should we do?

Well, when our coalition developed methodologies to treat chest pain, syncope, and sepsis, their consensus-written algorithms had to live somewhere for the doctor to conveniently use them. We decided to make them accessible on tablets or smartphones and to utilize data collection in the form of a QR Code Reader (a two-dimensional bar code, readable by smart phones) rather than paper forms that had to be laboriously completed and that got in the way of gaining true insight into why an element of the algorithm had been deviated from. If you type in the word "chest pain" or "syncope" or "sepsis," the QR code comes up. When the doctor scans it, the algorithm magically appears on the screen with a trunk-and-branch answering sequence to elaborate on variations.

We've mentioned that about 80 percent of medical teams will use the algorithm. The other 20 percent have good reasons not to use it. The QR reader allows them to share details about why they choose to *not* use it. With that information, we can make continuous adjustments to the algorithm, ensuring it is always on the leading edge of patient care. Even better, the medical staffs are inspired because their input is the catalyst for change.

On our journey to widespread transformation, we turned a barrier in the physician-patient relationship (the screen on a tablet or smartphone) into a benefit—a moonshot innovation.

The Patient Scores

Perhaps the most talked-about developments from our projects are the HEART score (for chest pain), the HEAD score (for syncope), and the NEWS2 score (for sepsis). Those were the focused moonshots derived from a synthetical approach. But one innovation branching out from those moonshots is most critical: linking those scores into the system through the electronic medical record. For the physicians and nurses, the algorithms are always top of mind—embedded in the culture of care.

The success of integrating those scores has spread into other areas. Now, an advanced imaging test can be used and ordered by the emergency physician (previously, it could only be ordered in the observation unit or inpatient unit). So, although we often view the EMR as a barrier to patient care, we found a way to convert the barrier into a powerful platform for change.

The Bigger Benefits of a Moonshot

After Neil Armstrong made history by being the first person to step foot on the moon in 1969, he looked back on the entire mission experience and gave a big-picture perspective:

> "This was a project in which everybody involved was, one, interested, two, dedicated, and three, fascinated by the job they were doing. And whenever you have those ingredients . . . you're going to win."

It's amazing to think it only took eight years after President Kennedy's moonshot speech for his vision to come true. The mission inspired everyone in the country to participate with either their heart, their head, or their hands. It wasn't about "trying." It was "doing." There's a big difference.

The grassroots change we've implemented in our local healthcare system hasn't taken much time at all. We don't need thousands of research papers and planning for decades. The changes are alive. We're using them. We're measuring them. We're receiving feedback and recirculating the methodology. Not quite instantaneously, but very quickly compared to the glacial movement of traditional methods and practices.

More important than all the tangible benefits are the intangibles: Unifying a diverse group of professionals into a common cause. Taking the high road over the righteous path. Committing to the right care at the right time with the right venue and right disposition for each patient—and appealing to our central passion to live a life of purpose.

> "This was a project in which everybody involved was, one, interested, two, dedicated, and three, fascinated by the job they were doing. And whenever you have those ingredients . . . you're going to win."
> —Astronaut Neil Armstrong

So when we quantified the clinical results of saving thousands of lives and millions of dollars, when we listed out the moonshot innovations and intangible benefits, and we presented those to the once-13-year-old boy who had gone to hear John F. Kennedy say, "Ask not what your country can do for you, but what you can do for your country," Dr. Moorhead said to us, "Wow, I wasn't expecting this."

He had given us perhaps the most powerful moonshot innovations of all—more important than technology, data gathering, even exploration: the freedom and trust to transform healthcare, not only in America, but everywhere, for generations to come.

With a shared purpose, anything is possible.

KEY POINTS FROM CHAPTER TEN

- **Barriers to transformation.** Longstanding protocols in healthcare can create barriers that make patient care less safe, effective, and timely than it should be. However, facing the barriers and finding ways to remove them paves the way for innovation and change.

- **Patient discharges.** The simple act of embedding a button into the ER's computer program made it easier to discharge patients with a follow-up appointment in place rather than holding them longer than necessary.

- **Dental emergencies.** We found a way for the ER to extend care in an innovative way for patients with dental emergencies.

- **QR readers.** We made the consensus-written algorithms accessible on the doctors' smartphone or tablet via QR codes to streamline care and record data to promote iteration.

- **Where the EMR fits.** Integrating the algorithms into the EMR makes them not only convenient but keeps them top of mind. The barrier of laborious record-keeping has become part of our platform for transformation.

- **Freedom and trust.** Having the freedom and trust to transform healthcare may be the most important innovation of all.

REFLECTIONS

- What barriers have you discovered as you implement your plan for transformed care?

- Write down those barriers. Challenge your coalition and frontline to think of ways to use the barriers to innovate solutions.

- What additional innovations would help implement your coalition's plan—with potential applications in other types of care? Think outside the box.

CHAPTER 11

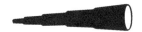

Earthquakes Are Coming

We Can Either Brace for Them or Break New Ground Ourselves

It seems like yesterday, October 17, 1989. I'm (Jeff) watching the pre-game show of the World Series between the San Francisco Giants and the Oakland As. Suddenly, I notice the TV camera starting to shake a little bit. At first, I just think it's a little strange. Then the picture goes fuzzy until *boom*, the screen goes completely black. When the broadcast returns, we're told a strong earthquake has shaken the Bay Area of California.

The earthquake triggers fires, collapses bridges, and crumbles homes. Nearly 4,000 people are injured, sixty-seven people die, and when all is said and done, the conservative estimate is at least $5 billion in damages throughout the area. The World Series itself is put on hold, postponed for 10 days. The Bay Area Earthquake measures 6.9 on the Richter scale and generates a variety of public reaction:

It could have been worse in such a heavily populated area.
Is there a bigger one coming?

Geologists have warned for decades about impending disaster along the fault lines in California—what are we doing about it?

Just five years later, in Southern California, disaster strikes along another fault line as an earthquake measuring 6.7 on the Richter scale hits the Northridge area. Apartment buildings collapse. Roads are destroyed. Gas mains break and force widespread evacuations. The economic impact is estimated at nearly $50 billion, making the Northridge Earthquake one of the costliest natural disasters ever. The heaviest toll, however, are the more than fifty lives lost and the thousands of injuries.

Scientists suggest these earthquakes are just a warning, leaving people to continually ask, "When will *the big one* hit?"

Fast-forward three decades to 2019. Toward the high desert region of Southern California, on the 4th of July, a series of strong earthquakes rolls through a swath of the state. The strongest one measures 7.1 on the Richter scale. Despite being much stronger than the Bay Area or Northside Earthquakes, overall damage is less severe, power outages are only sporadic, and no deaths are reported.

> With a shared purpose, anything is possible.

Why the vast difference in consequences?

Besides the obvious difference in the population density of the earthquake locations, there's also a difference in how structures and roads are engineered in the 25–30-year span. Every earthquake, even the minor activity, has posed a sobering reality that more earthquakes are coming, and at some point, an event far worse than anything experienced so far is very likely to happen. Government leaders and construction engineers could have dug in their heels and told everyone to brace themselves for the worst. But instead, with each passing year, they've proactively made changes based on input from those who see the damages and risks up close. Building codes are based on experiences rather than old standards. Roads and bridges are built with the likelihood of earthquakes in mind. Newer homes now have earthquake-resistant foundations and pipelines, and taller structures are developed with more flexibility to enable them to move when the earth moves.

There's still progress to be made, and yes, there's only so much you can do to mitigate the damages from a major earthquake. But rather than sticking with the status quo and hoping for the inevitable to never happen, Californians from the grassroots to the state capitol have made transformative decisions over the past twenty-five years to forge their own future rather than stand by and succumb to it.

Even while changes are being implemented, seismologists are recording small tremors by the dozens every week, serving as constant reminders of what could be coming . . . and perhaps as motivation to get ahead of it.

The Tremors in Healthcare

Those of us in healthcare feel like the residents of California who live near fault lines. We feel the tremors every day. We sense the warning signs of something major coming up. The healthcare structure as we know it cannot continue to be anchored on the same foundations we've rested on for a century, not while costs skyrocket and people die too soon. For the most part, the changes we've seen over the past thirty years—driven largely by insurance companies and government requirements—have had the effect of putting fresh coats of paint on a vulnerable structure and building a fence around it.

Meanwhile, we ask, "When will the big one strike and shake everything up?"

The reason Dr. Moorhead wanted us to explore new pathways for patient care is that we all knew the worst action we could take in the midst of the tremors is to wait. If we stand still and lean on rigid foundations—the protocols and processes that direct our work—then we're only ensuring that the damage from "the big one" will be disastrous. The infrastructure we've come to know for decades will not protect healthcare. And by "healthcare," we're talking about the heart of our purpose: the patient. The healthcare "big one?" A global pandemic? Are we prepared?

With that in mind we turned our attention from long-held standards to the people who work on our front lines—our greatest assets. Every day they experience the tremors in emergency departments and wherever the patients and their families are hurting. Our physicians and nurses are akin to the engineers who see the vulnerability of roads and buildings long before natural disasters strike. Who knows better than they how to improve care for patients?

The dramatic results we've described can be traced back to our willingness to embrace new pillars, starting with flexibility. With some flex in our approach to patient care, "the big one" in healthcare won't have such disastrous effects.

Our work is transformed, and we feel prepared for anything.

We Need a Big Earthquake

The healthcare landscape has been shaking for about thirty years. At the risk of sounding crazy and insensitive . . . maybe we *need* an all-out earthquake. Here's what we mean:

We tend to see two types of changes in healthcare—forest fires and glaciers.

The forest fire is quick. In our work this is the rapid-cycle improvement to show an immediate result. The change doesn't last, or at the very least it is not transformative. Think of how a forest fire scorches trees, bushes, and fields. Everything in the aftermath looks quite different . . . temporarily. We've seen the phenomenon in Florida, where the land is charred. Days later, literally, you see green sprouts in the barren landscape. The vegetation soon grows back. A forest fire doesn't permanently change the land. Disastrous as it might be, it is not transformative.

The glacier effects are all around us in healthcare. A glacier certainly changes the landscape, but it takes hundreds of years to move, scrape, melt, and form a final impression. And then the changed earth remains stagnant for a few more centuries. Just look at the basic model of a hospital. We treat patients in exchange for money. It's a business model that hasn't changed at all. Yes, the payment process has changed. More people and more institutions are involved in the transactions. But the system itself is old. We aren't saying payment for a service is wrong. But when the method of paying, and the amount being paid, becomes the focal point of healthcare . . . it's time to do something different.

And that brings us to the earthquake. It's drastic. It's sudden. It's a major shift, usually after many pre-shocks are felt. Sometimes it's anticipated; sometimes it isn't. The changes are permanent, and the aftershocks don't completely cease—they're subtle and persistent.

The harsh reality is this: An earthquake is coming to healthcare.

Time to Shake the Ground Ourselves

This is no time to take shelter and wait for an earthquake to happen. Neither do we need to wait for others to tell us how and when to respond. We can *make* it happen before the impending event itself.

In our hospitals, we've found one of the most effective ways to initiate earthquake-like transformation is to shift from the rigidness of evidence-based practice to the flexibility of practice-based evidence. Using one or the other alone is not in the best interest of patient care. Cookbook medicine isn't the be-all and end-all answer, and neither is care based on how a physician happens to feel about a condition on Tuesday. Our methodology blends the science and the art of medicine into synthetical decision making, which builds up the all-important pillar of flexibility.

The advantage of incorporating *some* evidence-based medicine is that it brings proven methods into the equation. The disadvantage is that evidence-based medicine is less personal. That's the beauty of practice-based evidence. It's mostly unwritten. Proper care is determined up close, one patient at a time. It includes the story of that person's life and utilizes that story in his or her care.

Physicians already know the medical journals inside and out, but they also bring lifetimes of experiences into patient care. We don't want them to feel beholden to distant and random clinical trials without consideration of their own personal input. The dogmatic approach in healthcare is like telling an engineer to use a certain foundation for a home in California because it's acceptable in Florida. In our methodology, optimum care hinges on how the frontline people observe those warm bodies—the patients who need healing.

So, in our method that's saved millions of dollars and thousands of lives, we allow for deviations. It's a big change for many hospital executives. At one stage in our implementation of the chest-pain methodology, an executive literally told us, "Just tell the physicians what to do."

It's good that he trusted us. But the trust wouldn't mean much if we hadn't convinced him to also trust the front line and to accept some variances and flexibility from traditional methods. He was obviously thinking in terms of a rapid-cycle improvement. Edicts from a front office might generate a temporary response, even a result. But if people on our front line reluctantly use our algorithms because they feel compelled to do so, well, we might as well chase after the wind. There will be no seismic paradigm shift. It just won't happen.

Breaking New Ground

English is the official language in the US and UK. But our uses of the same words can be worlds apart. Order "chips" in the US and you expect potato chips, but in the UK, you'll get french fries. Braces align teeth in the USA but hold your pants up in the UK—two nations divided by a common language.

We have language chasms in American hospitals, too. To the administrators, "risk" is associated with finances. To the physicians, risk is equated to a patient's well-being.

For us to be out in front of the forthcoming earthquake, we all need to be talking the same language with the same meaning. If the patient is truly the core of our work, then our conversations should reflect that. If we trust the physicians and nurses who are at the bedside day in and day out, then our decisions throughout healthcare will reflect that, too. In actionable terms, this means:

1. Empowering the frontline medical teams to help design the best methods for care
2. Removing obstacles they identify
3. Holding them accountable

Our collaborative methodologies with chest pain, syncope, and sepsis have saved money and lives. But the real transformation is the way physicians now treat each patient and how the hospital functions and flows. Patients are not lost in an abyss of data and technology. Physicians and nurses are more passionate about their purpose. The changes in our treatment of just three medical conditions have fostered dramatic change in the treatment of other diagnoses as well.

In other words, we've created our own purposeful tremors—and they're spreading. The landscape and the culture are different today.

So, yes, an earthquake *will* happen in healthcare. But it doesn't have to devastate us or paralyze us with concern. If we do nothing, we're doomed to suffer painful consequences that will reverberate through decades of aftershocks. However, if we prepare by reworking our foundational principles, strengthening our relationships, being more flexible, and focusing on patients rather than protocols, we'll be ready to handle the seismic shifts productively and confidently. We dare even say we might look at the prospect of an earthquake . . . *enthusiastically.*

KEY POINTS FROM CHAPTER ELEVEN

- **Everyday tremors in healthcare.** All of us that work in healthcare can feel the tremors and sense that something big is coming soon to shake up healthcare. Waiting is not an option.

- **The importance of flexibility.** Blending the science and the art of medicine into synthetical decision making builds up the all-important pillar of flexibility. Rigid structures will crumble, so we need to be willing to change now.

- **Practice-based evidence.** Focusing on practice-based evidence that allows for deviations creates a seismic paradigm shift in the way we practice healthcare.

- **Bridging our language chasms.** Frontline staff and front office administrators need to be talking the same language with the same meaning if we're to save lives and money.

- **A fearless approach to the future.** We can either wait for an earthquake to transform healthcare or we can create our own seismic transformation before the "big one" hits.

REFLECTIONS

- Ask your frontline team about the barriers that still remain.

- Write down the danger of *not* removing the barriers (how serious is the earthquake that could result from status quo)?

- Empower the team to create a plan to remove those barriers.

CHAPTER 12

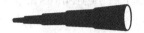

Heating Healthcare from the Bottom Up

A Handful of People Can Influence Thousands

Blue skies are not everyday sights in London. But one morning not long ago I walked out of my hotel room and felt this radiance from the sunlight all around. I (Danny) had traveled back to my home country for a conference of the Royal Society of Medicine (RSM), and you could say optimism was in the air. The RSM offers continuing medical education in the UK, and because its membership consists of providers and educators it has a solid reputation in the medical community. They were about to share insights from a group of national healthcare leaders who took on a mission to change a growing problem with antibiotic prescriptions. The promise of a good story about transformation in a healthcare system piqued my interest.

In the conference I heard how the NHS had become concerned that doctors had overprescribed antibiotics for years. Patients who came in with the slightest sniffle or sneeze were handed a script and, next thing you know, they had 10 days' worth of pills. The abundance of antibiotics meant people of all ages throughout the motherland were at risk. Overuse of antibiotics can encourage resistant bacteria to thrive. Over time, this had the potential to lead to a serious national health crisis. Recognizing this risk, the leaders wanted to change the doctors' behaviors toward prescribing antibiotics, and patients' physical responses to them. As I listened, I thought we might apply lessons from the "success story" to larger change—culturally and economically—anywhere in the world.

> It's amazing what happens when everyone can take credit, has a voice, participates, influences the pathway for patient care, and sees the results. The power is staggering.

Except this story didn't have a happily-ever-after ending—which is exactly the valuable takeaway.

These medical leaders wanted to warn general practitioners to carefully consider the ramifications from randomly following a systematic process of prescribing antibiotics. Their message, in essence, would be: "Stop conforming to an old protocol. Do what's best for each patient. Otherwise, we'll have a bigger problem."

They told us how they'd agreed to craft a letter to express this national concern. The content of the letter was, for the most part, on target. Over the course of a year, it altered the overall behavior toward antibiotic prescriptions, but only slightly. Prescriptions dropped by three percent—but still, maybe an early indication of a momentum swing in the right direction.

Then, whatever tempo had been gathering . . . stopped. Just like that, prescriptions returned to previous levels. What these leaders shared is another classic case of rapid-cycle improvement in healthcare with disappointing results.

The language of the message itself hadn't necessarily been the problem. The tires screeched because one high-ranking official signed the letter to be circulated to primary care doctors.

It appeared to be delivered from an imaginary marble-floored executive office. The message had a singular spokesperson . . . and zero chance of making a sustainable difference.

Doctors in the UK would have been far more likely to heed the advice in the letter had it come from trusted peers who treat sick patients every day—doctors just like them. With 20–20 hindsight, the group of healthcare leaders should have invited primary care physicians to engage in the process and to identify the barriers in limiting prescriptions. And then the physicians should have been allowed to craft the letter *and to sign it*. There's no telling how much traction the movement would have generated. Certainly, more than a 3 percent change that lasted all of one year.

Our Most Important Ambassadors

Change is just change until it's sustained. Sounds poetic. But it is so true. To sustain change, you need to identify an energy source and utilize it. That source becomes your flywheel, constantly moving the chain. Our flywheels in healthcare are the medical teams. This is why we invite doctors and nurses to be participants in the creation and implementation of pathways for care. They come up with reasonable measures to sustain the change. And guess who's held accountable to those measures? *They* are.

We witnessed how a groundswell of change can work—and then fall flat—at one hospital. Anesthesiologists there had developed a plan to reduce the number of surgery patients who needed to be on vents more than 24 hours. Sure enough, after being implemented, their design helped patients recover more quickly post-surgery—saving money and improving the patients' overall health. No one should have been surprised. Who would know the optimum way to administer anesthetics better than anesthesiologists?

But a problem arose soon after they started seeing results. Everything simply petered out. Why? Because the anesthesiologists weren't allowed to *lead* the change. They weren't empowered or given the flexibility to make adjustments as needed. The old ways of just knocking out patients for surgery crept back into their work. Today, those doctors share a story of frustration with nonsustainability of rapid-cycle improvement projects, but unfortunately no story of transformation.

If the front line isn't empowered to lead, then any effort to move forward will stall and retreat. We need physicians at the front of the train. And we need to realize they typically go through four phases before fully embracing major change:

1. "I don't believe your data."
2. "OK, I believe it, but my patients are different."
3. "I'll change when X changes." (The X-factor is usually "the hospital," "my colleagues," or "the government.")
4. "All right, let's do it."

It's crucial to bring them into the process rather than dictating it to them. When physicians and nurses feel fully invested, then everything can spin in the same direction. And it will keep spinning if those same frontline people are integral to creating, implementing, adjusting, and being accountable to the change at hand.

How We Fully Energize a Team

Attempting to change healthcare from the executive offices is the blowtorch tactic for heating a pot of water—you'll heat the surface but never break through to the rest of the pot. The front line is your fire-from-below. They create the bubbles that become bigger bubbles . . . until you have a full boil. When personable people who are trusted and respected lead the change, others will say, "All right, show me how we're going to do this."

We sensed a real shift early in our own pilot when a physician in our coalition told us about a 45-year-old patient who'd entered the hospital through the emergency department because of chest pain.

"She had some atypical symptoms, so instead of relying on my gut I actually followed the algorithm. The first blood test came back normal. But the algorithm we wrote said to wait three hours for the second blood test to come back. So I had to be patient and wait. Turns out, the second test showed an increase in her cardiac enzymes, indicating a problem with her heart muscle. We took her into treatment right away.

"The algorithm saved my butt and might have saved her life."

You don't hear doctors share stories with this kind of animation very often. This doctor was excited. He'd been involved in developing a method to treat chest pain. Then he used it himself. And he saw a woman's life change because of it. His passion became contagious.

A Few People Can Influence Thousands

We hear this question quite a bit: Who takes credit for saving lives and money, and for transforming a culture?

The answer: *Everyone*.

The boiling water is all of us. It starts with the coalition, a few enthused doctors and nurses who form those little bubbles rising from the bottom of the pot. They join together to make bigger bubbles until everything in the pot is hot. It's amazing what happens when everyone can take credit, has a voice, participates, influences the pathway for patient care, and sees the results. The power is staggering.

Those who use the practices of lean or Six Sigma often talk about the Deming Principle. They say if you want to influence 100 people, you use the square root to figure out how many influencers you need—which would be 10. You tell those ten people what kind of change you need, and they deliver the message.

But in the transformation principle, influencers from the front line are the very people who develop the idea and implement it. With this approach, you can reach far more employees with fewer influential people. It's remarkable. Instead of using a square root, you look at the cube root. So to transform a healthcare company of 24,000 employees, you need only 29 people. But not just any people. They have to be the *right* people who can naturally engage, empower, and become provocateurs of change.

POWER OF INFLUENCE	
DEMING PRINCIPLE $\sqrt{}$	TRANSFORMATION PRINCIPLE $\sqrt[3]{}$
⊙ Tell 10 people what to do. ⊙ They influence 100 people.	⊙ 29 people decide what should be done. ⊙ They influence 24,000 people.

The concept of transforming a healthcare organization isn't so ominous when we see it through that formula. You just need a few bubbles to rise up. Think of the people who to this day are the most influential in your life. It might be a parent or a sibling or a colleague. No doubt one reason you hold them in such high regard is trust. That person cares about you with no ulterior motive. Trust is the lifeblood of relationships, and it should be the lifeblood of healthcare. So the person your team trusts is the person you want on your coalition—the core of your cube root. The trust people have in him or her is the energy behind transformation.

Wrong Business Principles

Certain business concepts, when applied to healthcare, show a lack of trust. They cool the water that we work so hard to heat. For example, the phrase "failure is not an option" makes for a nice pre-game speech. Business leaders use it too. But the game-changers of today say the opposite. They're all about disruptive innovation, which seldom starts with a directive from the top to be perfect. Amazon heated the retail industry from the bottom. Southwest did the same with air travel, and Uber with ground transportation. They transformed their respective industries by taking journeys on paths rife with obstacles and lacking road signs. Do you think they experienced a few failures while they took risks? If we're to transform healthcare, we have to let it be known, *failure will happen along the way.*

Dr. Moorhead told us, "I'm not sure where this will take us, but let's see." Executive leadership fully supported us and what we were trying to do. They understood that venturing into new terrain meant there would be missteps while we identified obstacles, removed them, and readjusted as we moved forward. Because you cannot innovate if you're trying to perfect well-worn methods.

One huge obstacle we've faced in our journey to save lives and money is the hospital system itself. Yes, the electronic medical record can be a valuable tool when it's used for actual patient care, but nowadays we view it as an electronic *financial* record. The system makes it too easy to check a box and admit a patient instead of doing what's best. That's why we decided to ask the people at the bedside in simple language, "Put the electronic medical record and financial data aside. Forget the paths of least resistance. Just tell us what you do. *And tell us how we can empower you to do it better."*

That alone has been an epiphany. Start with a few people. They have all the resources we need. Their input. Their expertise. Their ideas. We don't need a big budget, lots of bodies, or the pomp and circumstance of fancy presentations. In short, the process comes down to three actions:

1. Determine where the problem is.
2. Identify the frontline influencers you want involved to solve it.
3. Follow them.

By doing that, we've seen fruits from our team's labor. And we've been reminded that a good harvest is not the result of thinking and waiting. It's from *doing*.

KEY POINTS FROM CHAPTER TWELVE

- **Creating momentum.** In order to sustain any change, it's important for trusted frontline medical teams to lead the way.

- **Reluctant physicians.** Physicians typically go through four stages before fully embracing major change. Knowing these four stages will help turn reluctance to buy-in.

- **Mobilizing a team.** Enthusiasm rises and change becomes permanent when everyone is given a voice, participates, sees results, and can take credit.

- **Staggering benefits of empowerment.** In the transformation principle, influencers from the front line are the ones who develop the idea *and* implement it. With this approach, you can reach far more employees with fewer influential people—29 people can influence 24,000 employees.

- **Failure *is* an option.** Innovations do not usually take place by staying within comfortable paradigms. The fear of failure will paralyze us from taking the risks necessary to transform healthcare. Failure *must* be an option.

- **Doing vs. thinking.** Transformation is not the result of thinking and waiting; it's from *doing*. Doing actively creates change, while thinking passively accepts the status quo.

REFLECTIONS

- Reassure the physicians and nurses that *they* are the leaders of this change.
- Publicly give credit to everyone who participates in the new methodology for patient care, especially as the successes are shared.
- Collect feedback and continually act on it to keep the cycle in motion and to generate enthusiasm.

CHAPTER 13

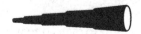

The Future Hospital... Today

From Doctor's Workshop to Focused Factory to Customized Care

Back in 1971 three really smart guys who had studied at the University of San Francisco decided to open a coffee shop in Seattle. These young men didn't really fit the existing mold for "corporate business leadership." They just loved coffee and tea, and they thought there were probably other people like them—maybe those people would be willing to pay a few cents more for a quality product served in a homey environment.

They were taking a big leap based on intuition.

At that time, and for the next 20 years, if you lived anywhere other than the Northwest US and you said you were "going out for coffee" it meant you headed to the convenience store on the corner. You poured your own coffee into a Styrofoam cup from a pot that had been warming all day—maybe since yesterday. You'd toss a quarter into a bowl and be on your way. The pot served dozens of people a basic product: coffee.

While those guys in Seattle were still reimagining the coffee business by listening to customers and observing their behaviors, a few food-and-beverage giants also saw an opportunity to increase revenue by selling coffee. McDonald's figured if they could sell billions of hamburgers, they could eventually sell billions of cups of coffee. They had a huge advantage over the corner store in terms of volume, resources, and efficiencies. They'd even pour the coffee for you! Soon, every fast food restaurant and every gas station in America would be selling coffee out of enormous tanks, quickly, and at a healthy profit.

By now you know the men who launched the coffee shop in Seattle were onto something all along: Starbucks. The corner-store coffee pot is a thing of the past. We can still go to McDonald's or Burger King or Chick-Fil-A and order the same cup of coffee that everyone else is served there. Or, we can go to a place like Starbucks. The brand those three guys founded is synonymous with customized coffees and teas. They had a vision for coffee 3.0 nearly 50 years ago. The barista asks each customer a few questions. You detail exactly what you want. And then they will literally personalize your coffee, right down to putting your name on the cup. It isn't their coffee anymore. It's *yours*.

The history of the way coffee is served reminds us of how we deliver healthcare to patients. It's a similar progression, leaving us on the cusp of what we see as the last of three phases:

Healthcare 1.0, The Doctor's Workshop

Through most of the 1900s, you could think of the hospital as a building with many tools. Doctors would come in and use the hospital as a place to conduct their work—surgery, childbirth, and urgent procedures. Patients would only go to the hospital for the type of care that couldn't be performed in the doctor's office. The hospital had the space and the resources for a doctor to do the serious part of their practice. The patient would put on a gown, lie on a bed, and the doctor would come and fix them up. Then the doctor would leave.

Healthcare 2.0, The Focused Factory

The work of doctors changed significantly toward the end of the 20th century. Insurance reimbursements and government requirements compelled healthcare providers to consider volume and time constraints. The pendulum swung hard in the direction of "efficiencies." Manufacturing processes and Six Sigma principles were implemented as the driving forces to make healthcare more productive and, more importantly, more profitable. The hospital turned into the focused factory with more tests, more data, and more protocols. The patient in the focused factory was treated as a product, or a widget.

Healthcare 3.0, Customized Care

This is the stage where we put the patient's name on the personalized cup. We've tried what supposedly works at the proverbial corner store and McDonald's. It's time to get back to what we love: making each patient better and healthier. To do that really well, we have to leave the doctor's workshop and the focused factory in the past. The best patient care doesn't always follow a linear path. It's active and alive. Customization means we empower frontline teams to use synthetical thinking—that blend of experience, firsthand evaluation, history, local data, and relationships. Then they can craft a pathway to healing and health for each patient—individually, personally, and wholistically.

We Are *in* the Future

When you mention football dynasties to even a modest fan, the reaction is either love or hate. We've had the Pittsburgh Steelers, the Dallas Cowboys, and the New England Patriots. Each was a polarizing team in their respective era because they won so many championships and they went about it in their own way. No matter how anyone felt about them, we can learn from the successes of teams like that.

Those teams didn't follow old football standards. Every pro football organization will say, "Neither do we," when in fact they all do, at least to some degree. But dynastic teams evaluate players differently. They proactively create a culture. They value consistency in a coach and in an on-field leader. As far as anyone can tell, they don't rely on formulas or hard-and-fast principles. Yes, they have a game plan every week. The coaches customize it to identify the obstacles they're likely to encounter from a particular opponent with input from their most respected players. But during an actual game, the frontline leaders have the freedom and confidence to make evaluations in the moment. The quarterbacks have the trust to adjust a play, called an "audible" in football. Those audibles are based on the situation, the factors they see in front of them, and past experiences they've tucked into the subconscious. In other words, the audible is a decision made from synthetical thinking.

> We won't deliver the best patient care possible if our medical teams are trained to stay the course and never deviate.

No one who desires the best result forces a quarterback who's won Super Bowls and has great relationships with teammates into a box by saying, "Forget what you see. Forget your experience. You need to follow the exact game plan we wrote up for you a week ago."

Neither will we deliver the best patient care possible if our medical teams are trained to stay the course and never deviate. The focused factory is the place where medical teams are bound to follow what everyone else is doing. Let's face it, even the most glowing optimist would say the results from the 2.0 model have not been great. We've become too dependent on technology to guide our work in the factory. Now we're even putting hope in artificial intelligence as the grand solution to our healthcare problems. While technology plays a role in customized care, the danger is being so infatuated with it that we lose touch with the patient.

> Do not confuse "advancement" or "high tech" with our ultimate goal: real transformation.

Do not confuse "advancement" or "high tech" with our ultimate goal: real transformation. They are not the same.

The 3.0 phase, customized care, is agile, adaptable, personal, and accepted. It's truly putting the patient first, not just because they happen to be in the room, but because *the patient is our purpose*. And who better to create a pathway to wellness than the physicians and nurses at the bed? They know the playbook. They have the relationship. They've developed mutual trust with the entire medical team and the administrators. *They* are the keys to customizing care in our next phase of healthcare 3.0.

The story of a surgeon meeting with his team in our hospital is one of many that epitomizes the meaning of customized care. They were concerned about a patient whose appendix risked rupturing. This well-respected surgeon said to the team: "We're not here to simply take an appendix out. The best care might happen to include taking it out. But our job is to care for this patient, completely."

That's agile, adaptable, personal, and accepted. It is what healthcare—*real* health and *real* care—is meant to be.

KEY POINTS FROM CHAPTER THIRTEEN

- **Doctor's workshop.** Early in the 20th century, the hospital model provided doctors the resources for certain medical procedures that could not be done in their own offices.

- **Focused factory.** Later in the 20th century, waves of change brought more volume, more regulations, and more costs. Patients were treated as products, or widgets.

- **Customized care.** The best patient care is active and alive. Today, it needs to be relational, rooted in synthetical thinking: a blend of experience, firsthand evaluation, history, local data, and relationships.

- **Four key transformation qualities.** Customized care is agile, adaptable, personal, and accepted, truly putting the patient first.

- **The greatest motivation.** The patient is our purpose. That is what *real* health and *real* care is meant to be.

REFLECTIONS

- Hold up "patient care" as the focal point of your purpose. Use reminders in communications, conversations, visual cues, and any discussions about the successes of your team's new plan.

CHAPTER 14

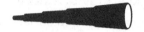

The Ultimate Question

Are You Ready to Transform Healthcare for Good?

I'll never forget the days leading up to the start of medical school. Specifically, I (Jeff) remember a sense of intimidation. *It's medical school. Lots of daunting goals and concepts. Complex formulas. Difficult applications.*

Like it is for many first-year med-school students, it's easy to lose focus in the stew of expectations.

Then, on my first day, the professors proceeded to teach me three things:

1. Listen to your patients. They'll tell you what's wrong with them.
2. Don't be overenamored by technology. Use it wisely or it will control you.
3. Give every patient something for their time of need.

They simplified medicine from a complicated universe of information and analysis to a basic action: Do what's best for the patient.

I thought, "*This* is why I want to be a doctor."

In the years since then, healthcare has gradually changed into what I had initially feared. Often, we seem to be working for a system rather than for a purpose. We follow protocols instead of listening to patients. Technology and data overwhelm our decision making. Analytical thinking has become highly valued while synthetical thinking is now considered cavalier. Complexities distract our focus from the basic act of caring for people in their time of need.

However, we can reclaim what we're passionate about. The reason we're so sure of it is because we're proving it right now in our own work.

At the start of this book, we made an ambitious and audacious promise: a path to truly transform healthcare. We wouldn't blame anyone for being skeptical. The idea of transformation is more intimidating than the start of medical school. But again, we're overthinking it. Because as the saying goes, "Simplicity is the ultimate sophistication."

Our transformation method is as simple as the three takeaways from that first day of medical school. In fact, the very first morning we discussed how to transform healthcare, we wrote down three musts:

1. Listen to the physicians. They'll tell you how to best care for patients.
2. Don't be overenamored with technology. As a whole, technology is a great tool . . . until it begins to control our decisions.
3. Give the medical team an algorithm to use when they need it. Even let them create it and adjust it.

Look at that list. If you're anything like us, it reminds you of why you wanted to get into healthcare in the first place.

Lessons from Mister Rogers

Fred Rogers always knew what people of all ages and backgrounds desired, even if we didn't know it ourselves. He created, wrote, and produced one of the most beloved children's shows of all time: *Mister Roger's Neighborhood*. The series ran for 33 years, won dozens of awards, and, nearly 20 years after the final episode, inspired a movie and a documentary that broke all-time records for gross revenue. In its heyday, the show riveted children. In its recent glory, it has brought adults to tears. As Joanne Rogers, Fred's wife of 50 years says, "We all long for what Fred represented."

Relationships. Caring. Simplicity. Those were the hallmarks of the man and of his show. Television executives often tried to nudge Fred Rogers into quickening the pace of his show, adding more colors and sounds, and including flashy visual effects. Fred's polite response: "No, thank you. The audience understands just fine."

He knew what we now know: More is not better.

And that's what we need to recapture in healthcare. Another pile of data won't take us where we need to go. Neither will a robotic system where policies overwhelm practice. If we're waiting for the next wave of technology to save healthcare, we're wasting our time. We could argue the hallmarks of healthcare echo those of Mister Rogers: Relationships. Caring. Simplicity.

The transformative methodology we've shared in this book really does direct us back to those qualities. Our medical teams have proven that it works. They're saving money ($32 million as of 2019 just in chest-pain treatment) and saving lives (a 63 percent decrease in the sepsis mortality rate over a two-year period).

But there's even more to it than sheer numbers—much more.

Now It's Your Turn

People ask us, "Do you have an individual patient story to crystalize the success of what you're doing?"

Our answer: "We have a quarter of a million patients with individual success stories. They've been shaped in only four short years, and for chest pain alone. The vast majority will tell you they were treated and not hospitalized. All of those who were discharged can talk about their experiences because none of them lost their lives due to being discharged."

There's a parallel story of victory that is equally important. It's the way these methodologies have revived the passion of medical teams. More than 120 physicians have been involved with patients presenting with chest pain in our emergency department. For sepsis, hundreds more physicians and nurses have followed a patient from the emergency department into the medical surgical ward, or the intensive care unit, and then back through the continuum of care.

One of our most experienced physician leaders, who's been practicing for more than twenty years, helped design the syncope algorithm. After the pilot, he said, "This has changed the way I care for patients."

An experienced medical director at one of our other hospitals helped design the sepsis algorithm. He said, "I finally get it. When I follow the algorithm and use the Sepsis Power Plan, it's like pulling a fire alarm to let everyone know that smoke has been detected. We're taking action instead of waiting to see if anyone actually gets burned from flames."

They're involved in it daily, firsthand. They will not go back to old ways. The culture is transformed. And it hasn't taken as long as you might think.

The transformation is even extending beyond the hospital. A member of our staff, but not on the clinical side, works part time in a large theme park. People get excited at the parks and forget to drink enough water in the Florida heat. They eat foods that, well, let's just say might not be the most nutritious choices. Sure enough, one day while this hospital employee was there, someone fainted. He told us later, "When I saw the person collapse, I rushed over, and you know the first thing I did? I utilized the HEAD score the medical team developed for syncope."

Right there in the park, someone who isn't even a physician or a nurse took what he'd learned from the hospital's culture and evaluated someone who was hurting. He had no data or technology to use—just the algorithm. He also had the freedom in that moment to think synthetically, whether he knew it or not. The park guest recovered after receiving the right care (paramedics) at the right time from a person who wanted to make them better in their time of need.

To be clear, we aren't saying this is the be-all, end-all plan for the future of healthcare. But it is a new direction. It's exciting. It's familiar. And it's far more effective than we ever would have believed when we started.

So, knowing all of this . . . now what do you do? A Christian will say the Bible is just a book unless you live it out. A doctor will say exercise is just an idea unless you actually do it. In the same way, our charge to you is summed up in a quote attributed to Thomas Edison, which says, "Vision without execution is just hallucination."

The vision is right here, with a game plan that anyone can execute. Dramatic change in healthcare is needed now. Inspiration is the spark, and motivation is the fire. Transformation will ignite the inferno to save money, save lives, and rekindle the passion of our medical teams. It will ultimately save healthcare.

KEY POINTS FROM CHAPTER FOURTEEN

- ◉ **A daily reminder.** This is why we wanted to be doctors and nurses in the first place: healing and health. We *can* reclaim what we're passionate about.

- ◉ **Decluttering healthcare.** The path to meaningful transformation is through simplicity and common sense.

- ◉ **The value of relationships.** They're at the heart of the best patient care—and now we know that relationships have tangible value, too, in both money and lives saved.

- ◉ **Success stories.** We have at least 250,000 patients who have benefited from transformed care in just a few hospitals. And that number represents only chest-pain patients.

- ◉ **The future is now.** Imagine if we all take charge and transform *all* healthcare together. What can you do to begin a transformation where you work?

REFLECTIONS

- ◉ Keep communicating. Keep engaging. Keep the momentum moving forward.

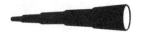

Epilogue

The first draft of this boo was written in 2019, covering the first five years of clinical transformation efforts at one hospital system. In 2020 when the world went on pause, our teams' work shifted to the phases of a global pandemic (prophetically forecast in chapter 11). Public health messaging and practices, workplace and PPE protection, different types of testing, new therapies and treatments, vaccination, and emergence of variants tested healthcare professionals and systems. Evidence-based practice was introduced more rapidly than in recorded history. Sharing practice-based evidence went national and international as fast as the respiratory virus. The "earthquake" that hit healthcare was a seismic shift that helped accelerate many advances in caring for patients. Telehealth, remote patient monitoring, hospital at home, and new vaccine development technologies are just a few of the needed advances. Danny and I (Jeff) engaged the frontline physicians caring for COVID patients in the emergency department, hospital wards, and intensive care units, as well as in ambulatory and post-acute units. The methodology described in this book led to the *Guide to COVID Care*, first published and distributed in August of 2020 to forty U.S. hospitals. Periodic updates, based on evidence and practice with input from those doing the lifesaving care every day, are available to physicians and nurses via QR code, EMR, or web access.

As important as being laser-focused on COVID was, we were interested in knowing how the other transformational efforts were faring. After all, if they were just rapid cycle improvements, the successes may have been transient. To our relief, they not only continued, but the measures showed even more improvement. When you change the culture, the improvements are permanent and become "the way we have always done it."

Ready For More?

Bonus Material to Take You Further

Now that you've read *Transformative Healthcare*, there are additional bonus materials for you at the book's website: TransformativeHealthcareBook.com. When you sign up for the publisher's newsletter, you will get access to free bonus materials, such as:

One-Page Summary: A summary of the *Transformative Healthcare* highlights on a single page that you can print out, refer to often, and share with others.

Author Recommendations: Dr. Kuhlman and Daniel Peach have gathered a list of recommended books and resources for additional insights around *Transformative Healthcare.*

COVID-19 Care Non-ICU Protocol: The methodology described in *Transformative Healthcare* led to the *Guide to COVID Care*, first published and distributed in August of 2020 to forty U.S. hospitals. Included online is the most recent COVID-19 Non-ICU Protocol. Care protocols are rapidly changing as new information comes to light and the most recent version is posted online.

Secrets to Growing Physician Leaders: Learn how physicians can become better leaders and discover how to motivate others and "lead up" in this guide from a retired US Army Lt. General and leadership teacher.

14 Secrets to Healthcare Leadership: Hospital leaders are tasked with minimizing costs, upholding metrics, and accomplishing the mission. All while providing overall direction. In this guide, you'll discover how to get your clinical staff and executive staff working in harmony towards the same goals.

And even more: Find even more resources expanding on change management, synthetical thinking, medical models, and healthcare innovation.

Sign up now at **TransformativeHealthcareBook.com**

Appendix

Research Paper

EClinicalMedicine 10 (2019) 78-83

Published by *The Lancet*

Clinical Transformation Through Change Management Case Study: Chest Pain in the Emergency Department

Jeffrey Kuhlman, David Moorhead, Joyce Kerpchar, Daniel J. Peach, Sarfraz Ahmad, Paul B. O'Brien

Clinical Transformation, AdventHealth Orlando, Orlando, FL 32804, USA

ARTICLE INFO

Article history:
Received 1 November 2018
Received in revised form 12 April 2019
Accepted 16 April 2019

Keywords:
- ED
- SCAMPs
- Chest pain
- Heart score
- Clinical transformation
- Change management
- Physician behavior and practice
- Reduction in cost and resource utilization

ABSTRACT

Introduction/Background: Adults with chest pain presenting to an emergency department are high-risk and high volume. A methodology which gathers practicing physicians together to review evidence and share practice experience to formulate a written algorithm with key decision points and measures is discussed with implementation, based on change management principles, and results.

Methods: A methodology was followed to "establish the standard-of-care". Literature and data were reviewed, a written consensus algorithm was designed with ability to track adherence and deviations. We performed a before and after analysis of a performance improvement intervention in adult patients with undifferentiated chest pain in our nine-campus hospital system in Florida between January 1st, 2014 and December 31st, 2018.

Results: A total of 200,691 patients were identified as adults with chest pain and the algorithm was used. A dramatic change in the disposition decision rate was noted. When the 'Baseline-Year' was compared with the 'Performance-Year', chest pain patients discharged from the ED increased by 99%, those going to the 'Observation' status decreased by 20%, and inpatient admissions decreased by 63% (p b 0.0001). All patients were tracked for 30-days for major adverse cardiac event (MACE) or return to the ED within the same system. If the s emergency physicians had not changed their practice/behavior and the Baseline-Year decision rate during the entire Performance-Year was unchanged, then 4563 more patients would have gone to Observation and 7986 patients to Inpatient. The opportunity costs avoided would be approximately $31million (US$).

Conclusions: For successful clinical transformation through change management, we learned: select strategic topics, get active physicians together, write a consensus algorithm with freedom to deviate, identify and remove barriers, communicate vision, pilot with feedback, implement, sustain by "hard wiring" into the electronic medical record and measure outputs.

---

*Correspondence to: J. Kuhlman, AdventHealth-Orlando, FL 32804, USA.
**Correspondence to: S. Ahmad, AdventHealth Medical Group, 2501 North Orange
Avenue, Suite 786, Orlando, FL 32804, USA.
E-mail addresses: jeffrey.kuhlman@AdventHealth.com
(J. Kuhlman), sarfraz.ahmad@AdventHealth.com (S. Ahmad).

https://doi.org/10.1016/j.eclinm.2019.04.010
2589-5370/© 2019 Published by Elsevier Ltd. This is an open access article under the CC BY-NC-ND license (http://creativecommons.org/licenses/by-nc-nd/4.0/).
Contents lists available at ScienceDirect
EClinicalMedicine EClinicalMedicine 10 (2019) 78–83

journal homepage: https://www.journals.elsevier.com/eclinicalmedicine
© 2019 Published by Elsevier Ltd. This is an open access article under the CC BY-NC-ND license (http://creativecommons.org/licenses/by-nc-nd/4.0/).

1. Introduction

Chest pain is one of the most common reasons for presentation to the emergency department (ED). Chest pain represents 5–10% of adult ED visits, however less than 1% of cases need acute intervention [1]. Clinical difficulty lies in identifying patients with acute coronary syndrome (ACS) needing prompt intervention from those that do not.

Mismanagement of ACS in the ED is a top medical-legal issue. The diagnosis of ACS is missed in approximately 2% leading to substantial consequences, including a short-term two-fold increase in mortality for patients with acute myocardial infarction (MI) who are mistakenly discharged from the ED. [2]. For patients at low risk of ACS these concerns must be balanced against the cost and inconvenience of tests, procedures or admission, for individuals with low probability of improving the ability to discriminate patients with or without active cardiac ischemia or to improve patients' outcomes.

In 2014, AdventHealth (formerly Florida Hospital) became a founding partner of the Institute for Relevant Clinical Data Analytics (IRCDA), an organization who developed the Standardized Clinical Assessment and Management Plans (SCAMPs) methodology to improve patient outcomes while reducing practice variation and unnecessary resource utilization [3]. SCAMPs provide a better alternative to clinical practice guidelines [4] and are a preferred methodology to incorporate evidence-based medicine into practice and may fit better in the culture of medicine, obtaining clinician adoption and better influence the clinical decision making [5]. SCAMPs offer a pragmatic and well-accepted methodology to standardize practice, optimizing resource use while improving patient care [6–10].

AdventHealth (formerly Florida Hospital) with their nine geographic campuses under a single hospital license had 414,005 adult ED patient visits during the year 2014. The chief complaint with the highest volume, highest risk, and highest variability was undifferentiated chest pain or angina with 28,324 adult patients with a final primary or secondary diagnosis of R07.2, R07.89, R07.9, I120.0, I120.1, I120.8 or I120.9 (Table 1).

A Clinical Transformation department was established. Inspired by the SCAMPs methodology, adapted from change management principles,11 an AdventHealth Clinical Transformation (ACT) method was conceived and implemented (Fig. 1).

2. Materials and Methods

A guiding team of emergency medicine physicians, cardiologists, and nursing leadership was assembled representing an influential coalition. A vision to "establish the standard of care" for this patient population was developed and communicated. Following the ACT methodology, the pertinent systematic review of chest pain risk stratification was performed, current data was presented, a consensus algorithm (adapted from three SCAMPs pilots at Brigham and Women's Hospital; 10/14/ 2012 to 5/20/2014) was drafted (Fig. 2) with plans to capture the data from adherence to and deviations from the algorithm.

During the planning process, four critical components emerged as essential elements to algorithm formation:

i. **Identification:** Adults with undifferentiated chest pain presenting to the ED.

ii. **Indications:** Inclusions: Chest discomfort/pain, chest pressure/fullness, pain radiating to left/both arms, jaw pain, pain in back/neck/stomach, shortness of breath, cold sweats, nausea/vomiting, lightheadedness. Exclusions: High concern for ACS on presentation [patients with STEMI (ST segment elevation myocardial infarction), definite NSTEMI, heart failure, arrhythmia, or non-cardiac etiology such as gastrointestinal, musculoskeletal or pulmonary.

iii. **Stratification:** The HEART (History, EKG, Age, Risk factors, Troponin) score was chosen as the best stratification tool. The HEART score [12,13] had been prospectively validated for ED chest pain patients in The Netherlands via risk stratification with significantly higher concordance (c-statistic) than the Thrombolysis in Myocardial Infarction (TIMI) or the Global Registry of Acute Coronary Events (GRACE) scores. A secondary analysis of the Myeloperoxidase in the Diagnosis of Acute coronary syndromes Study (MIDAS) at 18 tertiary referral centers in the United States showed the HEART score identified a substantial number of low-risk patients for the early discharge, by incorporating a serial troponin measure, while maintaining high sensitivity for ACS [14].

iv. **Actions:** Patients in the low-risk category (HEART score 0–3) would have a repeat troponin blood test in three hours and if normal would be discharged with cardiology or primary care physician follow-up within 72 h. Patients in the intermediate risk category (HEART score 4–6) were recommended for observation status. Patients with a high-risk for ACS (HEART score 7–10) were recommended to be admitted for further evaluation and treatment.

After the consensus algorithm was defined, obstacles and barriers were identified (and mitigated):

- Lack of ability of "low-risk" patients to get an appointment with primary care physician or cardiologist within 72 h of ED visit. (Establishment of care coordination center able to make outpatient appointments, before patient even left the ED)
- Assurance of fairness: Patients with the established medical staff relationship return to their physician, unassigned patients (payor agnostic) to primary care physician (PCP) or non-interventional cardiologist on call for the campus ED. (Adherence to medical staff by-laws and utilization of the campus call schedule)
- Need for feedback to emergency physicians regarding the appointment compliance and 30-day outcomes of those transitioned to outpatient follow-up. (ACT team provided monthly report)
- Concern regarding shifting the medical-legal risk from in the hospital to the doctors' offices. (Discussion and education)
- Concern regarding shifting the financial burden of self-pay patients from the hospital to doctors' offices. (Awareness of hotline for scheduling follow-up for 45-days after the ED visit with hospital covering self-pay or narrow network patients)

Research in context

Evidence Before This Study

The research team reviewed the world literature in reference to chest pain risk stratification tools. The search terms included stratification of undifferentiated chest pain in the emergency department and run through PubMed. The body of evidence supported the use of HEART Score as an internationally accepted risk stratification tool.

Added Value of This Study

This study shows that clinician compliance to an evidence-based protocol can be sustained when coupled with a hospital supported outpatient care navigation platform. This conclusion is important as previous papers have suggested poor ability to sustain compliance to an outpatient chest pain algorithm.

Implication of All the Available Evidence

The results to this study point to the importance of a reliable process when a patient is transitioning to the outpatient care setting from an acute care setting. Emergency physicians may be able to implement more complex algorithms if there is timed accountable follow-up. Interestingly, an evidence-based algorithm is enough to foster compliance unless it is coupled with a population health mechanism. As healthcare goals are more focused on cost, quality and utilization, safe patient management outside the hospital becomes a priority. Future research on physician compliance with evidence-based algorithms other than chest pain, such as syncope and abdominal pain may benefit from the model highlighted in this paper.

The pilot was submitted for our Institutional Review Board (IRB) vetting and it was determined this study was classified by the IRB as a "performance improvement initiative and not human subject research". A 400-patient pilot was planned at a 398-bed hospital for two months, June–July of 2015.

Table 1

Chest pain/angina definitions by the ICD-10a.
ICD-10

R07.2 Precordial pain
R07.89 Other chest pain
R07.9 Chest pain, unspecified
I120.0 Unstable angina
I120.1 Angina pectoris with documented spasm
I120.8 Other forms of angina pectoris
I120.9 Angina pectoris, unspecified

Abbreviations: ICD=international classification of diseases; ACT=AdventHealth Clinical Transformation
[a] Patients receiving an emergent cardiac intervention were excluded from the study set as accorded by the algorithm.

2.1. Lessons Learned from the Pilot

From the pilot study, we learned the following:

i. Many physicians voiced opposition to "recipe medicine", but no clinician disagreed with the consensus algorithm.
ii. Communication with the physicians (emergency medicine, primary care, cardiologists) is never enough, and needs to be done in many venues.
iii. An electronic order needed to be created in the electronic medical record (EMR) for the call coordination center to reach into a physician's office schedule and make a follow-up appointment for a patient while still in the ED.
iv. The hospital has a "45-day tail" and phone hotline for any patient who was discharged from the ED to receive any pertinent testing ordered by the PCP or cardiologist, and costs are covered by the hospital.
v. Patients identified as "low-risk" were more appropriate for primary care follow-up to address modifiable risk factors vice cardiologists. vi) The "ACT effect" was felt, as the emergency medicine physicians would, on occasion, use the algorithm follow-up on patients they were caring for, whether they were ACT patients or not.
vi. The "hard wiring" of the HEART score into the emergency physicians electronic work flow is critical for the maintenance and sustainment of the effort.

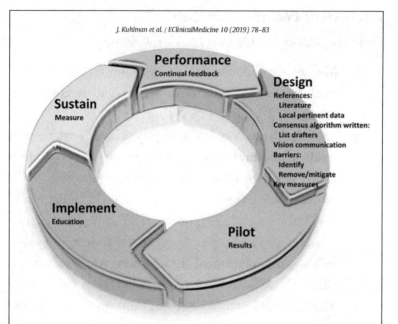

Fig. 1. AdventHealth Clinical Transformation (ACT) cycle.

Design
- Demonstrate change needed now (evidence, data)
- Assemble guiding team, powerful coalition of active clinicians (written consensus algorithm)
- Develop motivating vision (best for patient)
- Communicate vision (urgency, honesty, clarity, passion)
- Identify and remove/mitigate barriers/obstacles (key measures)

Pilot
- Short run win (results, deviations, iterate)

Implement
- Maintain focus, build (education)

Sustain
- Institutionalize into culture (behaviors, attitudes, processes, ongoing measures)

Performance
- Continual feedback

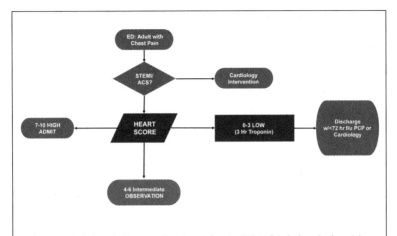

Fig. 2. *High level chest pain algorithm*. *This high-level algorithm is an abridged version of the full interdisciplinary algorithm.*

2.2. Full Implementation

Results and lessons learned from the pilot were presented and discussed with the entire healthcare system cardiologists and emergency medicine physicians. Unanimous approval was given to implement it system-wide, which was done campus by campus in the fall of 2015.

2.3. Maintenance and Spread

Every emergency medicine department and the core physicians' meetings were attended by the Clinical Transformation leaders, and physicians were educated on the ACT process, including a visit to all the cardiologists' offices.

2.4. Process Measures/Data Collection

Data were collected and reported to the ED leaders for evaluation, which included:

i. The number of forms completed by the emergency physician (to assess adoption and need to education).
ii. Follow-up on the number of patients in ACT algorithm.
iii. The HEART score distribution.
iv. Appointment recommended (no-show/decline vs. attend).
v. Re-visit status of patients who received/recommended appointments when discharged from the ED.

The ACT algorithm was fully implemented on November 1, 2015. The HEART score was "hard wired in the EMR" on December 7, 2015. Full system-wide implementation was completed on January 1, 2016 with monthly feedback of appointments and the HEART score use by the individual physicians.

> **Table 2**
>
> Performance of change management stages during the design/pilot years implementation.
>
> Adults ED
>
> 2014 Y0 — Baseline
> 2015 Y1 — Design/pilot
> 2016 Y2 — Implement
> 2017 Y3 — Sustain
> 2018 Y4 — Performance
>
> Chest Pain 28,324 37,903 41,640 44,057 48,767
> Total 414,005 441,932 480,110 502,109 511,395
> 6.8% 8.6% 8.7% 8.8% 9.5%
>
> Abbreviations: ED — emergency department; Y = year.

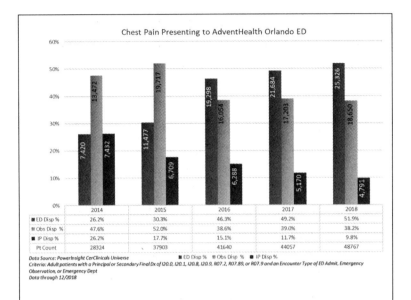

Fig. 3. Patient count and Disposition Decision Rate Breakdown for adults with chest pain/angina presenting to the emergency department from January 1, 2014 to Dec 31, 2018.

3. Statistical Analyses

We performed statistical tests and CI (confidence interval) using "Two Proportions" method. We also used matching and stratification to deal with any confounding effect. p-Values b0.05 were considered statistically significant.

4. Results

During the design/pilot, implement, sustain and the performance years, 200,691 patients were identified as adults with chest pain and the algorithm was used (Table 2). A dramatic change in the disposition decision rate was noted. When the 'Baseline Year' was compared with the 'Performance Year', chest pain patients discharged from the ED increased by 98% (26.2% to 51.9%), p b 0.0001), those going to the 'Observation' status decreased by 20% (47.6% to 38.2%; p b 0.0001) and 'Inpatient' admissions decreased by 62.5% (26.2% to 9.8%); p b 0.0001) (Fig. 3).

All ACT patients were tracked for 30-days for major adverse cardiac event (MACE) or return to the ED within the same healthcare system. Of the 40,791 patients identified as "low-risk" during the implement and sustain years (2016–2017), three cases returned within 30-days with MACE. A retrospective blinded review by a senior emergency medicine physician re-scored all three cases as "intermediate-risk" on the initial presentation and observation status would have been more appropriate. Refresher training was provided to all the emergency medicine physicians. Limitations to the study population include patients with 30-day MACE presenting to a hospital outside of our system or on the Social Security Death Index were not available. Limitations to the study also included the subjective nature inherent in one parameter of the HEART score.

Our findings were consistent with a contemporaneous multi-center study [15],which determined that "in adult patients with chest pain admitted with two negative findings for serial biomarkers, non-concerning vital signs, and non-ischemic electrocardiogram(EKG) findings, short-term clinically relevant adverse cardiac events were rare and commonly iatrogenic, suggesting routine inpatient admission may not be beneficial strategy for this group".

5. Discussion

Many strategic initiatives are attempted in healthcare, often with initial success [11,16] A more sustaining approach to changing the behavior and practice of physicians is by engaging physicians to design the care algorithm, track the data, embed decision making tools in the EMR, and encourage deviation for individual patient variation. ACT is an innovative method of examining relevant clinical data to improve patient outcomes while reducing practice variation and unnecessary resource utilization.

Our experience utilizing the ACT algorithm for patients with chest pain in the ED suggests that the percentage of patients identified as "low-risk" and safely transitioned to outpatient appointment for the continued evaluation and treatment nearly doubled while patients going to an observation decreased. Those found requiring inpatient admission were more than cut in half. By "hard-wiring", the HEART score in the EMR and vigilantly monitoring the process measures (appointments and the HEART score utilization) by individual physician, the clinical change needed to improve the care of adults with chest pain presenting to an ED was maintained and sustained.

The change management approach enabled Emergency Physicians to develop an algorithm based on evidence and practice experience. The process and the results when communicated back to the physicians facilitated them to change their behaviors and practices to safely identify the appropriate venue to take care of adults with chest pain presenting to the emergency department. Equally important to the study was the continued maintenance (sustain) which had been a failing point in other studies to date.

In healthcare, the stroke of the pen (click of the mouse) is the determinant with the most powerful effect on cost of care. The difference in direct costs for a patient with ED discharge versus inpatient admission is US $3000 more for the admitted patient, with a final primary or secondary diagnosis of R07.2, R07.89, R07.9, I120.0, I120.1, I120.8 or I120.9. For Observation status, US $1500 more in direct costs is noted, compared to ED discharge [17].

An exercise of hypothetical analysis helps quantify the impact of the decision process (Table 3). If the Emergency Physicians had not changed their practice or behavior and the Baseline Year decision rate during the entire Performance year was unchanged, then 4563 more patients would have gone to Observation status and 7986 patients to Inpatient admissions. The one-year opportunity costs avoided would be approximately US $7 million (M) and $24M, respectively, for a total of $31M.

Reduction in bed use in the healthcare system with chronic overcapacity is also important. If one assumes 1.5 days hospital length-of-stay (LOS) for observation and 4-days LOS for inpatient, then a 19-bed observation unit and 88-bed inpatient unit would have been utilized. The "capital redirection" for optimized utilization could be hypothesized at US $100 M.

Table 3

Decision rate comparison, baseline to performance.

	Y0 Baseline	Y4 Performance	Y4 Performance Y4 if Y0 Decision rate		Y4 if Y0 Decision rate
ED to home	26.2%	51.9%	25,326	26.2%	12,777
Observation	47.6%	38.2%	18,650	47.6%	23,213
Inpatient admit	26.2%	9.8%	4791	26.2%	12,777

Reduced Observation annualized patients by 4563 ≥ $7M US$.

Reduced Inpatient Admits annualized patients by 7986 ≥ $24M US$.

Opportunity to save $31M US direct costs.

380 fewer Observation stays per month.

666 fewer Admissions per month.

More importantly than the cost and utilization exercise are the intersecting premises of transformation and safety. The human story of methodically identifying an additional one in four adult patients with chest pain who can safely be further evaluated in the outpatient setting meets the quadruple aim of the improved outcomes, lower cost, higher satisfaction, and improved experience for the healthcare team [18].

6. Conclusions

As healthcare continually strives to be fiscally responsible while maintaining patient safety, it is becoming increasingly important to identify patients that can be cared for in low-cost environments outside the hospital. This paper suggests that the safe disposition of undifferentiated chest pain presenting to the emergency room can be accomplished using the HEART Score coupled with a supportive outpatient infrastructure. We have successfully shown the ability to change emergency physician behavior and the ability to sustain the outpatient disposition rate in contrast to recent studies [13,19,20]. Our primary addition to the HEART score stratification was a hospital supported care navigation pathway that guaranteed all patients a 72 h follow-up with a PCP. The inference here is that emergency physicians will support and sustain outpatient discharge of low-risk patients as long as the outpatient hand-off is structured, timely, and set at the time of ED discharge. This has important implications for other outpatient diagnostic pathways that have a readily identifiable low-risk population.

Lessons learned for successful clinical transformation through change management

- Select strategic topics
- Get active physicians together
- Write a consensus algorithm with freedom to deviate
- Identify barriers and remove obstacles
- Communicate vision
- Mandatory pilot and transparent feedback
- Phased system implementation
- Sustain by "hard wiring" EMR, and outputs

Authors' Contributions

Dr. Jeffrey Kulhman: Conceived the study design and its implementation, performed literature search, data review and analyses, data interpretation, and manuscript writing.

Dr. David Moorhead: Discussed the study design and oversaw the project operation, and participated in data review, interpretation, and manuscript writing.

Ms. Joyce Kerpchar: Discussed the study design, participated in the project implementation and data review, interpretation and analyses.

Mr. Daniel J. Peach: Help conceived the study design and its implementation, performed literature search, data review, analyses, and interpretation, created figures, and writing.

Dr. Sarfraz Ahmad: Performed peer-reviewed literature search, scientific discussion, data interpretation, created tables, writing and preparation of the manuscript for publication.

Dr. Paul B. O'Brian: Help conceived the study design and its implementation in emergency medicine, performed literature search, data review, analyses, interpretation, and writing.

Conflict of Interest Statements

All the authors declare that there are no conflicts of interest associated with this research manuscript.

Role of Funding Source

None to disclose.

Ethics Committee Approval

This study was deemed exempt by our AdventHealth Institutional Review Board (IRB), and no patient consent was required.

Appendix A. Supplementary data

Supplementary data to this article can be found online at https://doi.org/10.1016/j.eclinm.2019.04.010.

References

[1] Mozaffarian D, Benjamin EJ, Go AS, et al. Heart disease and stroke statistics-2015 update: a report from the American Heart Association. Circulation 2015;131:e29–322.

[2] Mehta RH, Eagle KA. Missed diagnoses of acute coronary syndromes in the emergency room — continuing challenges. N Engl J Med 2000;342:1207–10.

[3] Rathod RH. SCAMPs: a new tool for an old problem. J Hosp Med 2015;10:633–6.

[4] Farias M, Jenkins K, Lock J, et al. Standardized clinical assessment and management plans (SCAMPs) provide a better alternative to clinical practice guidelines. Health Aff 2013;32:911–20.

[5] Farias M, Ziniel S, Rathod RH, et al. Provider attitudes toward standardized clinical assessment and management plans (SCAMPs). Congenit Heart Dis 2011;6:558–65.

[6] FariasM, Friedman KG, Lock JE, Newburger JW, Rathod RH. Differentiating standardized clinical assessment and management plans from clinical practice guidelines. Acad Med 2015;90:1002.

[7] Angoff GH, Kane DA, Giddins N, Paris YM, Moran AM, Tantengco V, et al. Regional implementation of a pediatric cardiology chest pain guideline using SCAMPs methodology. Pediatrics 2013;132(4):e1010–7.

[8] Friedman KG, Kane DA, Rathod RH, Renaud A, FariasM, Geggel R, et al. Management of pediatric chest pain using a standardized assessment and management plan. Pediatrics 2011;128(2):239–45.

[9] Moodie DS. Outcomes research-standardized clinical assessment and management plans. Congenit Heart Dis 2010;5(4):337.

[10] Sox H, Stewart W. Algorithms, clinical practice guidelines, and standardized clinical assessment and management plans: evidence-based patient management standards in evolution. Acad Med 2015;90(2):129–32.

[11] Kotter JP. Leading change: why transformation efforts fail. Harv Bus Rev 2007:11 January 1.

[12] Backus BE, Six AJ, Kelder JC, et al. A prospective validation of the HEART score for chest pain patients at the emergency department. Int J Cardiol 2013;168:2153–8.

[13] Poldervaart JM, Reitsma JB, Backus BE, et al. Effect of using the HEART score in patients with chest pain in the emergency department: a stepped-wedge, cluster randomized trial. Ann Intern Med 2017;166:689–97.

[14] Mahler SA, Miller CD, Hollander JE, et al. Identifying patients for early discharge: performance of decision rules among patients with acute chest pain. Int J Cardiol 2013; 168:795–802.

[15] Weinstock MB, Weingart S, Orth F, et al. Risk for clinically relevant adverse cardiac events in patients with chest pain at hospital admission. JAMA Intern Med 2015; 175:1207–12.

[16] Creasey T. Harnessing the power of change-enabling systems. Prosci®. https://www. prosci.com/resources/articles/harnessing-the-power-of-change-enabling-systems, Accessed date: 3 March 2019.

[17] Budryk Z. Two midnight rule means complications for hospitals, patients. Fierce Healthcare; 2014 July 15.

[18] Bodenheimer T, Sinsky C. From triple to quadruple aim: care of the patient requires care of the provider. Ann Fam Med 2014;12:573–6.

[19] Than MP, Pickering JW, Dryden JM, et al. Improving care processes for patients with suspected acute coronary syndrome (ICare-ACS): a study of cross-system implementation of a national clinical pathway. Circulation 2018;137:354–63.

[20] Kwong RY, Schussheim AE, Rekhraj S, Aletras AH, Geller N, Davis J, et al. Detecting acute coronary syndrome in the emergency department with cardiac magnetic resonance imaging. Circulation 2003;107(4):531–7.

Acknowledgments

Dr. Jeffrey Kuhlman and Daniel J. Peach

The authors must confess, any change to healthcare is achieved by the men and women in the arena. The frontline doctors, nurses, and advanced practice clinicians carry the burden of caring for patients every day. Our job is to support and empower them. Without their tireless leadership and contribution, nothing changes. We are forever indebted to the efforts of the many physicians and nurses at AdventHealth.

Our team, who thinks about and puts into action the change, innovation, disruption, and transformation so desperately needed in healthcare, includes Josh Lopez, Shelley Lanier, Michael Kuhlman, James Gershon, Angie Gentile, Christina Moreno, and Angela Victor. Their daily dedication inspires us, and they have our eternal gratitude.

Putting the concepts into tangible print, paper, and electrons could not have been achieved without the professionalism and persistence of the publishing team. Our editors, Todd Chobotar and Denise Putt, along with the rest of the AdventHealth Press team—Lillian Boyd, Sheila Draper, Danica Eylenstein, and Caryn McCleskey—are the essence of this book's existence. Robert Stephens made the stories impactful while deftly connecting the fabric of the concepts into the written word. They have our utmost thanks.

Special thanks to our peer reviewers, Allan Frankel, Louis Pizano, Joyce Kerpchar, and Piotr Kulach, who provided important insights and suggestions about our manuscript to make it even stronger and more compelling. The time, energy, and expertise they brought to the task is much appreciated.

Our penultimate thanks go to those who inspired us to consider a better way for improving healthcare. Jim Lock for pointing out that physicians hold the key to change based on their practice and experience coupled with evidence on occasion. Dave Moorhead, with his vision of having clinicians lead, reaping benefits from empowering them, working with them, and engaging with them for a lasting relationship based on trust and respect, has been a constant fountain of inspiration and perspiration.

Dr. Jeffrey Kuhlman

On the journey of life there is one individual who leads, follows, or walks alongside, providing guidance, encouragement, course correction, or unwavering support. Sandy Montaperto Kuhlman is my person, partner, and provider. Without her, there are no achievements in life. Thank you, Sandy!

Daniel J. Peach

I have been lucky to be blessed with the strength and support of my wife, Cheryl Peach, and children, Courtney and Shelley. Their light and energy help to enlighten me and, coupled with the strength of a family far away in miles but close in heart, give the guidance and will to always look up.

About the Authors

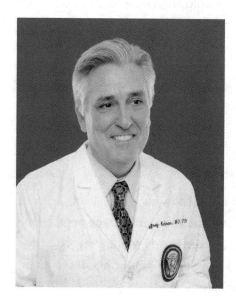

Jeffrey Kuhlman served as a navy physician for 30 years, 16 years supporting the White House physician to Presidents Clinton, Bush, and Obama. As the director of the White House Medical Unit, White House physician, and senior flight surgeon for Marine One, Kuhlman was required to be no farther than two minutes from the president at all times. In this role, he gleaned personal lessons about the importance of individual, relational care.

As physician to the president, Dr. Kuhlman coordinated comprehensive healthcare for the president and the first family, oversaw medical care for the vice president (and family) and for senior White House staff and Cabinet rank members. He was also responsible for emergency medical actions and advanced contingency planning, which necessitated the collaboration of the White House Medical Unit with the Secret Service protection details. Dr. Kuhlman provided guidance and advice on all joint service, interagency, and international matters for medical contingency planning and operations. He traveled to more than 90 countries to review their healthcare resources and protocols. His oversight even extended over force protection (preventive measures to mitigate hostile actions involving personnel, resources, facilities, and critical information), population health, and workplace health and safety programs for all workers and guests on the White House complex at home and abroad.

His mantra: "No policy. No politics. Just trusted medical advice."

Dr. Kuhlman is triple board-certified in aerospace, family, and occupational medicine. He's board-certified in medical management and a certified physician executive by the American Association of Physician Leaders and a certified professional in patient safety. His global health expertise includes the certificate in traveler health by the International Society of Travel Medicine. Currently, Dr. Kuhlman serves as chief quality and safety officer for America's largest Protestant not-for-profit healthcare system, AdventHealth, guiding quality, risk, safety, and transformation.

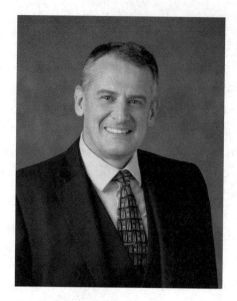

Daniel J. Peach serves as director of clinical transformation at AdventHealth Orlando, America's largest hospital. Since 2002, Peach, a registered osteopath in the United Kingdom, has specialized in prevention, care, and the optimization of human performance for elite athletes. During his 26 years in executive leadership for an international fiber-optic telecommunications manufacturer, Peach directed teams tasked with solving challenges of the people, processes, and technology interfaces. His work has included sensitive international security issues, where the safety of frontline and executive personnel requires high-performing leadership and action in real time.

HEAR MORE FROM
Dr. Jeff Kuhlman and Daniel Peach

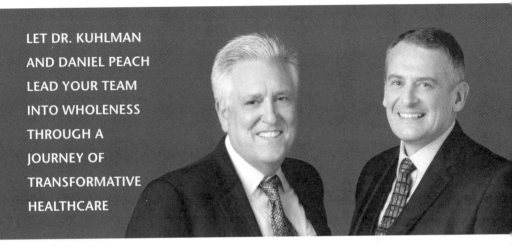

LET DR. KUHLMAN AND DANIEL PEACH LEAD YOUR TEAM INTO WHOLENESS THROUGH A JOURNEY OF TRANSFORMATIVE HEALTHCARE

The Authors Speak on Many Topics Including:

Jeff and Daniel
- **Transformative Healthcare:**
  How to Save Thousands of Lives and Millions of Dollars
- **Synthetical Thinking:**
  Unleashing the Most Powerful but Rarely Used Type of Thinking

Jeff
- **Presidential Healthcare in the 21st Century:**
  Lessons from a Decade as White House Physician
- **Protective Medicine:**
  Strategies for 24/7 Care During Domestic and International Movements

Daniel
- **Disruptive Innovation:**
  The Campfire Approach to Making the Change
- **Clinical Pathway Development:**
  Integrating Clinical Evidence to Arrive at a Consensus-Based Solution

To book Dr. Jeff Kuhlman and Daniel Peach
or another speaker for your event, visit:

AdventHealthPress.com

ABOUT THE PUBLISHER

AdventHealth is a connected network of care that promotes hope and healing through individualized care that touches the body, mind and spirit to help you feel whole. Our hospitals and care sites across the country are united by one mission: Extending the Healing Ministry of Christ. This faith-based mission guides our skilled and compassionate caregivers to provide expert care that leads the nation in quality, safety, and patient satisfaction.

Over 5 million people visit AdventHealth each year at our award-winning hospitals, physician practices, outpatient clinics, skilled nursing facilities, home health agencies and hospice centers to experience wholistic care for any stage of life and health.

AdventHealth Press publishes content rooted in wholistic health principles to help you feel whole through a variety of physical, emotional, and spiritual wellness resources.

To learn more visit AdventHealthPress.com.

RECOGNITIONS

CLINICAL EXCELLENCE. AdventHealth hospital campuses have been recognized in the top five percent of hospitals in the nation for clinical excellence by Healthgrades. We believe that spiritual and emotional care, along with high-quality clinical care, combine to create the best outcome for our patients.

TOP SAFETY RATINGS. We care for you like we would care for our own loved ones — with compassion and a priority of safety. AdventHealth's hospitals have received grade "A" safety ratings from The Leapfrog Group, the only national rating agency that evaluates how well hospitals protect patients from medical errors, infections, accidents, and injuries.

SPECIALIZED CARE. For over ten years, AdventHealth hospitals have been recognized by U.S. News & World Report as "One of America's Best Hospitals" for clinical specialties such as: Cardiology and Heart Surgery, Orthopedics, Neurology and Neuroscience, Urology, Gynecology, Gastroenterology and GI Surgery, Diabetes and Endocrinology, Pulmonology, Nephrology, and Geriatrics.

AWARD-WINNING TEAM CULTURE. Becker's Hospital Review has recognized AdventHealth as a Top Place to Work in Healthcare based on diversity, team engagement and professional growth. AdventHealth has also been awarded for fostering an engaged workforce, meaning our teams are equipped and empowered in their work as they provide skilled and compassionate care.

WIRED FOR THE FUTURE. The American Hospital Association recognized AdventHealth as a "Most Wired" health system for using the latest technology and innovations to provide cutting-edge, connected care.

PARTNERSHIPS

WALT DISNEY WORLD. AdventHealth has partnered with the Walt Disney World® Resort for over 25 years. As the Official Medical Provider for runDisney and Official Athletic Training Team of ESPN Wide World of Sports, AdventHealth has played a critical role in enhancing the Disney Parks and Resort operations and experiences for athletes.

In 2011, AdventHealth and Disney opened the Walt Disney Pavilion at AdventHealth for Children, which is now one of the premier children's hospitals in the nation, setting standards for innovation, quality and comprehensive care. The child-centric healing environment is designed to keep kids comfortable is complemented by a staff of world-class doctors, specialists, nurses and healthcare professionals utilizing advanced technologies, therapies and treatments. AdventHealth also collaborated with Disney to create AdventHealth Celebration, a cutting-edge comprehensive health facility that was named the "Hospital of the Future" by the *Wall Street Journal*.

STRATEGIC SPORTS. AdventHealth's commitment to whole-athlete care and innovative care models extends throughout our strategic sports partnerships, which span across multiple professional sports leagues including NBA, NFL, NHL, and NASCAR. AdventHealth is the Official Health Care Provider of the Orlando Magic, Lakeland Magic, Orlando Solar Bears, and Sebring International Raceway, Exclusive Hospital of the Tampa Bay Buccaneers, Official Health and Wellness Partner of the Tampa Bay Lightning, as well as the Official Health Care Partner and a Founding Partner of the iconic Daytona International Speedway.

In addition, through our 20+ year partnership with Florida Citrus Sports, AdventHealth has provided comprehensive health care services to collegiate athletes as the Official Health Care Provider for the Cheez-It Bowl and Vrbo Citrus Bowl.

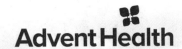

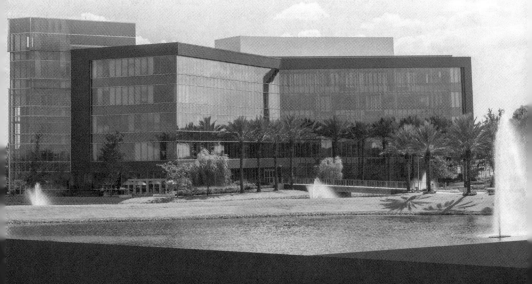

About AdventHealth Clinical

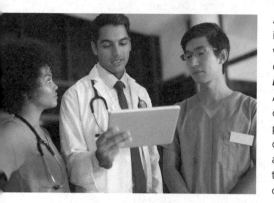

AdventHealth Clinical's strategic aspiration is for AdventHealth to deliver **world-class**, whole-person, clinical care with uncommon compassion consistent with our mission of **Extending the Healing Ministry of Christ**. A foundational **culture** of collaboration, communication, and transparency will provide the platform from which we will deliver this **exceptional** whole-person care as we lead in safety and clinical **excellence** through aligned systems, seamlessly connected networks, and shared strategies.

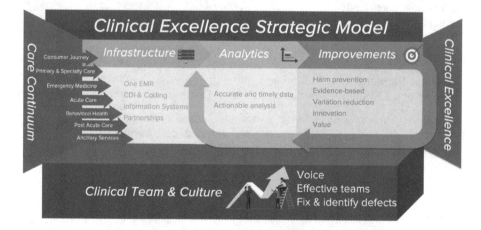

AdventHealth Clinical's **Clinical Excellence Strategic Model** empowers the company to focus on key strategies necessary to compete in a healthcare industry that is rapidly changing. To provide exceptional care to our patients we will need to:

- **Infrastructure:** Standardize documentation and coding practices to support providers and accurately and completely reflect the care and condition of the patient.
- **Analytics:** Create accurate, timely, and actionable data and analysis for superior decision-making.
- **Improvement:** Develop and implement clinical care strategies that drive safe, timely, effective, efficient, patient-centered, and equitable whole-person care.
- **Empower Clinical Workforce:** Using accelerated learning, technology, and optimized practices, build a world-class clinical workforce where the team members have a voice and proactively identify and fix defects.

The Measure of Success for AdventHealth Clinical is ensuring every AdventHealth facility has a 4- or 5-CMS Star Rating, an "A" Leapfrog Hospital Safety Grade, a top-quartile All Adult Inpatient Mortality, and a measurable reduction in harm.

AdventHealth Clinical supports a multitude of clinical programs:

Clinical Documentation/ Coding	Clinical Analytics	Performance Improvement
Quality & Safety	Safety Culture	Medication Safety
Imaging Safety	Unit Culture	Infection Prevention
Care Reliability	Clinical Innovation	Clinical Finance
Behavioral Health	Critical Care	Emergency Medicine
Medical Library	Nursing Leadership	Nursing Practice/Education
Care Management	Hospital Medicine	Healthcare Disparities
Ancillary Services	Research	

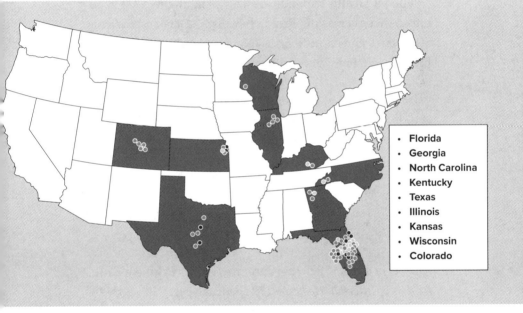

- Florida
- Georgia
- North Carolina
- Kentucky
- Texas
- Illinois
- Kansas
- Wisconsin
- Colorado

AdventHealth Clinical is located at the AdventHealth Corporate Headquarters in Altamonte Springs, Florida. AdventHealth Clinical supports 9 states across the United States.

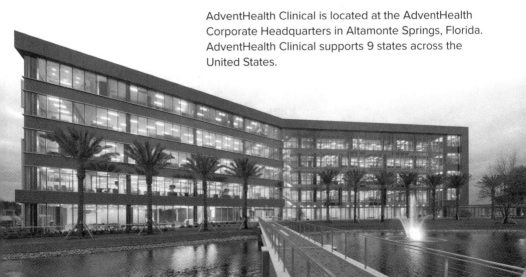

Endnotes

1. "National Health Expenditures 2017 Highlights," CMS.gov, https://www.cms.gov/Research-Statistics-Data-and-Systems/Statistics-Trends-and-Reports/NationalHealthExpendData/Downloads/highlights.pdf.

2. "The World Factbook – Country Comparison: Life Expectancy at Birth," CIA.gov, https://www.cia.gov/library/publications/the-world-factbook/rankorder/2102rank.html.

3. David U. Himmelstein et al., "Medical Bankruptcy: Still Common Despite the Affordable Care Act," *American Journal of Public Health* 109, no. 3 (March 1, 2019): 431–433, https://doi.org/10.2105/AJPH.2018.304901.

4. Kimberly Rask, "Pricing Patients Out of Primary Care," *Annals of Internal Medicine* 172 (February 4, 2020): 283–284, https://www.doi.org/10.7326/M19-4000.

5. Sorin T. Teich and Fady F. Faddoul, "Lean Management —The Journey from Toyota to Healthcare," *Rambam Maimonides Medical Journal* 4, no. 2 (April 2013): 1–9.

6. Institute for Healthcare Improvement Innovation Series, *Going Lean in Health Care*, Cambridge, MA: Institute for Healthcare Improvement; 2005. Available on www.IHI.org.

7. James P. Womack and Daniel T. Jones, *Lean Thinking: Banish Waste and Create Wealth in Your Corporation* (New York: Free Press, 2003).

8. From the Patient Safety & Quality Healthcare website—"http://www.psgh.com."

9. Kristina E. Rudd et al., "Global, Regional, and National Sepsis Incidence and Mortality, 1990–2017: Analysis for the Global Burden of Disease Study," *The Lancet* 395, no. 10219 (January 18, 2020): 200–211, https://doi.org/10.1016/S0140-6736(19)32989-7.

10. Unpublished Harvard study presented to Florida Hospital, 2014.

11. Mark H. Ebell et al., "How Good Is the Evidence to Support Primary Care Practice?" *BMJ Evidence-Based Medicine* 22, no. 3 (June 2017): 88–92, http://dx.doi.org/10.1136/ebmed-2017-110704.

12. Massachusetts Medical Society, Massachusetts Health and Hospital Association, Harvard T.H. Chan School of Public Health, Harvard Global Health Institute, *A Crisis in Health Care: A Call to Action on Physician Burnout* (Waltham, MA: Massachusetts Medical Society; 2018). Available on www.MassMed.org.

Index

A

Air Force One 5, 8, 9, 10, 11, 17, 20, 63, 78

Algorithm ix, 62, 63, 64, 65, 66, 67, 68, 69, 70, 71, 73, 83, 84, 86, 94, 95, 96, 100, 102, 103, 104, 105, 108, 109, 110, 111, 112, 113, 116, 118, 126, 131, 132, 134, 139, 140, 150, 168, 181, 183, 184, 191, 192, 194, 196, 197, 198, 199, 200, 201, 202, 203, 204, 205, 208, 210

  Chest pain 197, 201

  Consensus-written 62, 63, 66, 113, 149, 153

  Syncope 183

Antibiotics 42, 44, 121, 122, 123, 147, 148, 164, 165

Armstrong, Neil 151

B

Barriers 21, 65, 76, 79, 103, 104, 111, 112, 113, 144, 145, 146, 153, 154, 163, 166, 192, 196, 200, 208

Beijing 75, 76, 79

Bryant, Coach Paul (Bear) 108, 112

Button 118, 120, 121, 125, 145, 146, 147, 153

  Magic 120, 125

C

Cath lab 60, 132, 134

Change management 57, 58, 71, 73, 189, 190, 191, 192, 194, 202, 205, 207
   Principles 73, 191, 194
Chest pain xvii, 2, 9, 10, 12, 20, 51, 54, 55, 56, 60, 62, 63, 65, 68, 70, 71, 72, 73, 83, 84, 104, 105, 110, 115, 116, 117, 118, 124, 125, 131, 132, 133, 135, 136, 137, 140, 149, 150, 162, 168, 183, 190, 191, 194, 195, 197, 198, 201, 202, 203, 204, 205, 207, 210, 211
China 75, 79, 83
CIA 14
Cloud 94
Coalition 57, 59, 61, 62, 64, 65, 66, 96, 102, 103, 104, 107, 108, 110, 111, 112, 113, 115, 116, 117, 118, 119, 120, 125, 126, 134, 139, 141, 149, 154, 168, 170, 194, 200
Consensus-Written Algorithm 64
Consultants 31, 32, 34, 36, 49, 50, 51
Coronary Artery Bypass Graft (CABG) 46, 47, 48, 49, 50
   Pilot 48
   Trial 46, 49, 50
Culture change 33, 36
Customized care xviii, 174, 176

D

Data ii, iv, vi, 6, 13, 14, 16, 17, 18, 19, 20, 21, 22, 24, 25, 26, 27, 28, 30, 31, 32, 33, 34, 36, 39, 40, 42, 44, 46, 47, 48, 49, 53, 54, 55, 56, 57, 58, 61, 62, 66, 68, 79, 82, 86, 89, 90, 92, 93, 94, 96, 98, 106, 117, 149, 152, 153, 162, 167, 171, 176, 179, 181, 182, 184, 191, 193, 194, 200, 202, 204, 205, 208, 209

Administrators v, viii, 6, 7, 17, 19, 26, 52, 58, 85, 107, 135, 161, 163, 178

Clinicians iv, 17, 19, 32, 33, 52, 61, 67, 122, 200, 212, 213

Deming Principle 169

Dental kit 145, 147, 148

Design xiv, 3, 29, 56, 58, 59, 101, 102, 103, 104, 106, 107, 109, 110, 112, 162, 166, 183, 200, 202, 203, 204, 208, 209

Deviation 41, 64, 204

Discharge 60, 66, 67, 73, 103, 119, 120, 121, 133, 134, 138, 146, 147, 153, 195, 205, 207, 211

Button 145, 146

Patient 138

Dragonfly 114, 115, 123

E

Earthquake 155, 156, 157, 158, 159, 160, 161, 162, 163, 186

In healthcare 158, 162

Edison, Thomas 184

Electronic medical record (EMT) i, v, 19, 68, 104, 117, 120, 129, 150, 170, 171, 192, 199

F

Front line xv, 28, 33, 45, 54, 55, 73, 107, 109, 111, 112, 115, 124, 125, 126, 139, 161, 167, 169, 172

Empower/empowering the 41, 115, 125, 126, 162, 169, 171, 176, 212

Listen/listening to the 45

H

Harvard study 53

HEAD score 118

Heads in beds 129, 135, 140

Healthcare i, ii, iii, iv, v, vi, vii, viii, ix, xiv, xv, xviii, 1, 3, 4, 5, 6, 7, 11, 12, 13, 14, 16, 18, 19, 20, 21, 22, 25, 26, 27, 28, 29, 30, 31, 32, 33, 34, 36, 39, 44, 45, 46, 49, 50, 51, 52, 53, 54, 57, 58, 59, 61, 65, 66, 67, 68, 69, 71, 72, 73, 75, 76, 79, 80, 81, 82, 83, 84, 85, 86, 88, 89, 90, 91, 93, 94, 96, 97, 101, 102, 103, 106, 114, 115, 121, 123, 124, 127, 128, 131, 132, 135, 136, 138, 139, 140, 142, 144, 145, 146, 147, 148, 149, 151, 152, 153, 157, 158, 159, 160, 161, 162, 163, 164, 165, 166, 167, 169, 170, 172, 175, 176, 178, 180, 181, 182, 184, 185, 186, 188, 189, 197, 201, 204, 205, 206, 207, 211, 212, 213

Effective 25, 36

Expensive 7, 14, 16, 21, 36, 42, 49, 50, 51, 54, 55, 95, 117

HEART score 68, 84, 104, 105, 110, 117, 118, 123, 124, 125, 132, 150, 195, 199, 202, 204, 205, 207, 210, 211

I

Implement i, 6, 7, 20, 26, 30, 36, 56, 58, 59, 101, 106, 107, 108, 110, 123, 126, 154, 169, 172, 192, 197, 200, 201, 202, 203, 204

Improvements, rapid cycle 187

Influencers 169, 171, 172

Innovation i, ii, vii, 56, 57, 69, 119, 142, 146, 150, 153, 170, 189, 212

K

Kennedy, President John F. 142, 143, 144, 151, 152
Kotter, John 57

L

Leading Change 58
Lean ii, 26, 27, 28, 30, 40, 46, 49, 68, 70, 89, 90, 158, 169
  Manufacturing 27
  Thinking 28
Life expectancy 14, 15, 19

M

Methodology 20, 44, 54, 55, 63, 67, 68, 69, 70, 73, 77, 83, 85, 102, 105, 106, 108, 111, 112, 116, 118, 120, 125, 126, 131, 133, 135, 136, 139, 146, 151, 160, 161, 173, 182, 186, 188, 191, 193, 194, 210
  For chest pain 63, 70
  For sepsis 139
  For syncope 120
Metrics 32, 40, 54, 65, 91, 104, 189
Moonshot innovation 142, 144, 150

N

NEWS2 score 122, 123, 124, 150

O

Olympics 76

P

Pilot 9, 44, 48, 54, 56, 58, 59, 60, 66, 71, 72, 101, 104, 106, 109, 110, 134, 135, 139, 140, 168, 183, 192, 198, 199, 200, 201, 202, 203, 208

Practice-based evidence iii, vii, 53, 160, 163, 186

Protocol 9, 43, 79, 145, 165, 188, 197

Q

QR 145, 148, 149, 150, 153, 187
  Code 149
  Reader 149

R

Relationship ii, iv, v, ix, xiv, 8, 11, 18, 31, 36, 80, 83, 92, 117, 147, 149, 150, 178, 196, 213
  Administrator-clinician 18
  Doctor-patient ii, 18, 36

Rogers, Fred 182
  Mister 182

S

Sepsis 40, 41, 42, 43, 44, 49, 50, 83, 115, 121, 122, 123, 124, 125, 135, 137, 139, 140, 149, 150, 162, 182, 183
  Power Plan 122, 123, 124, 125, 139, 140, 183
  Trial 40, 50

Six Sigma 27, 30, 46, 70, 169, 176

Statistics 87, 88, 91, 92, 93, 96, 209

STEMI 60, 195

Strategy xvii, 37, 38, 48, 57, 59, 62, 65, 140, 204

Sustain iv, 35, 40, 41, 56, 58, 59, 67, 69, 101, 108, 109, 110, 134, 166, 172, 192, 197, 200, 202, 203, 204, 205, 207, 208

Syncope 115, 118, 119, 120, 121, 124, 125, 149, 150, 162, 183, 184, 197

T

Technology ii, iv, v, vi, viii, ix, 6, 7, 9, 14, 16, 18, 19, 20, 21, 22, 24, 25, 26, 28, 31, 32, 34, 69, 79, 81, 82, 83, 86, 94, 98, 107, 117, 128, 142, 152, 162, 178, 180, 181, 182, 184

The Lancet 20, 70, 71, 73, 190

Thinking i, ii, iii, iv, vii, xvii, 2, 3, 9, 11, 18, 19, 21, 24, 28, 30, 32, 56, 87, 88, 90, 92, 94, 95, 96, 97, 98, 99, 101, 113, 115, 116, 118, 126, 128, 132, 134, 147, 161, 171, 172, 176, 177, 179, 181, 189

  Analytical 88, 96, 132

  Five types of 88, 90, 98

  Synthetical iii, vii, 18, 19, 21, 24, 30, 92, 94, 96, 97, 98, 113, 126, 128, 134, 176, 177, 179, 181, 189

    Ingredients of 96

Tiananmen Square 77, 78, 79

Toyota 27, 28, 29

Transformation iii, iv, xviii, 3, 6, 19, 26, 28, 29, 30, 31, 34, 35, 36, 39, 41, 45, 50, 51, 52, 59, 64, 68, 71, 72, 99, 105, 110, 111, 112, 114, 115, 116, 118, 120, 121, 124, 125, 127, 139, 145, 150, 153, 160, 162, 163, 164, 167, 169, 170, 172, 178,

179, 181, 184, 185, 186, 190, 191, 192, 194, 198, 200, 201, 207, 210, 212

Transformative vi, 6, 11, 27, 32, 34, 40, 49, 71, 104, 106, 113, 115, 131, 157, 159, 182

Tremors 157, 158, 162, 163

V

Vision 57, 59, 62, 64, 65, 71, 103, 104, 112, 113, 115, 126, 147, 151, 175, 184, 192, 194, 200, 208, 213

W

Whole-person health 7, 137, 146, 234

Widgets xvii, 22, 27, 28, 36, 179

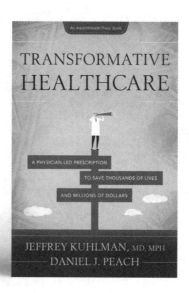

REGISTER THIS NEW BOOK

Visit AdventHealthPress.com

Benefits of Registering:

FREE **replacement** of lost or damaged book

FREE **audiobook** — *CREATION Life Discovery*

FREE information about new titles and **giveaways**

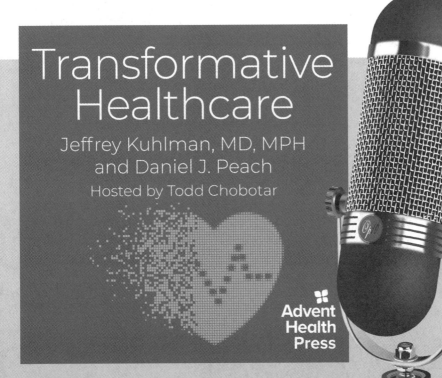

LIVE LIFE TO THE FULLEST

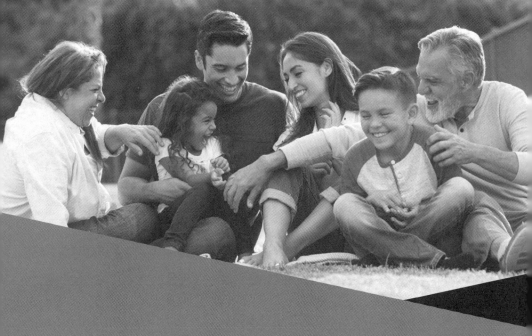

CREATION Life is a faith-based wellness plan for those who want to live healthier and happier lives and share this unique, whole-person health philosophy. By consistently practicing the principles of CREATION Life, we fulfill God's original plan for our lives, which is to live and be happy!

Our mission is to help you live life to the fullest, but we don't stop there. Feeling great is a feeling worth sharing, and we have the tools and resources to equip you for a health ministry.

Visit us at **CREATIONLife.com**
to get started on your journey to feeling whole!

ADDITIONAL RESOURCES

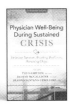

Physician Well-Being During Sustained Crisis
Discover support for clinicians who deal daily with long hours, stressful situations, challenging decisions and moral dilemmas. Learn from seasoned healthcare professionals working at the front lines as they tell their stories and offer counsel based on real-life experience.

Whole By His Grace
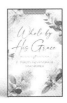
Whole by His Grace was written by women sharing the real struggles, triumphs, and lessons they have learned to inspire you with hope and courage as you face each day. Start each day with a story of hope or finish your day with a sense of His wholeness.

CREATION Health Breakthrough
Blending science and lifestyle recommendations, Monica Reed, MD, prescribes eight essentials that will help reverse harmful health habits and prevent disease. Discover how intentional choices, rest, environment, activity, trust, relationships, outlook, and nutrition can put a person on the road to wellness.

Pain Free For Life
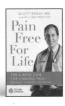
In *Pain Free For Life,* Scott C. Brady, MD, — founder of Florida Hospital's Brady Institute for Health — leads pain-racked readers to a pain-free life using powerful mind-body-spirit strategies — where more than 80 percent of his chronic-pain patients have achieved 80–100 percent pain relief within weeks.

Scalpel Moments
A scalpel moment can be one of painful awareness, disturbing clarity, sorrowful regret. It can also be a moment of positive awakening that can reveal, restore, and renew. Ordained minister Dr. Reaves highlights stories about life's difficult or revealing moments that remove layers of confusion, bitterness, or fear and restore one's trust in God.

The Love Fight
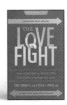
Are you going to fight for love or against each other? The authors illustrate how this common encounter can create a mutually satisfying relationship. Their expertise will walk you through the scrimmage between those who want to accomplish and those who want to relate.

AdventHealthPress.com

ADDITIONAL RESOURCES

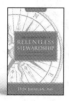

The Hidden Power of Relentless Stewardship
Dr. Jernigan shows how an organization's culture can be molded to create high performance at every level, fulfilling mission and vision, while wisely utilizing - or stewarding - the limited resources of time, money, and energy.

Leadership in the Crucible of Work
What is the first and most important work of a leader? (The answer may surprise you.) In *Leadership in the Crucible of Work,* noted speaker, poet, and college president Dr. Sandy Shugart takes readers on an unforgettable journey to the heart of what it means to become an authentic leader.

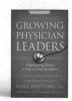

Growing Physician Leaders
Retired Army Lieutenant General Mark Hertling applies his four decades of military leadership to the work of healthcare, resulting in a profoundly constructive and practical book with the power to reshape and re-energize any healthcare organization in America today.

Bible Promises to Feel Whole
The Bible is packed with promises on health and healing - from aging to nutrition to rest, from grief to anger to stress. The *Bible Promises to Feel Whole book* collects over 600 scriptures in more than thirty different translations in a convenient pocket size on these topics and more including the CREATION Life principles.

SuperSized Kids
In *SuperSized Kids: How to Rescue Your Child from The Obesity Threat,* Walt Larimore, MD, and Sherri Flynt, MPH, RD, LD, explains step by step, how parents can work to avert the coming childhood obesity crisis by taking control of the weight challenges facing every member of their family.

Simply Healthy: The Art of Eating Well – Diabetes Edition
Simple, enticing, delectable, the recipes in *Simply Healthy: The Art of Eating Well – Diabetes Edition* will convince even the most skeptical that your food can taste good AND be good for you!

AdventHealthPress.com

ADDITIONAL RESOURCES

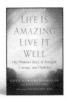

Life Is Amazing Live It Well
At its heart, Linda's captivating account chronicles the struggle to reconcile her three dreams of experiencing life as a "normal woman" with the tough realities of her medical condition. Her journey is punctuated with insights that are at times humorous, painful, provocative, and life-affirming.

Forgive To Live
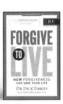

In *Forgive To Live: How Forgiveness Can Save Your Life,* Dr. Tibbits presents the scientifically proven steps for forgiveness — taken from the first clinical study of its kind conducted by Stanford University and Florida Hospital.

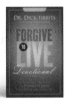

Forgive To Live Devotional
In his powerful new devotional Dr. Dick Tibbits reveals the secret to forgiveness. This compassionate devotional is a stirring look at the true meaning of forgiveness. Each of the 56 spiritual insights includes motivational Scripture, an inspirational prayer, and two thought-provoking questions. The insights are designed to encourage your journey as you begin to *Forgive to Live*.

Eat Plants, Feel Whole
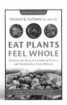

For over thirty years, Dr. Guthrie has been helping his patients gain better health through an evidence-based, whole-food, plant-based lifestyle. Now, in *Eat Plants, Feel Whole,* he shares not only his years of expertise with you, but the scientific evidence to back it up as well.

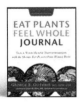

Eat Plants Feel Whole Journal
Everything you need to succeed with the *18-day Eat Plants Feel Whole* Plan. The companion journal is an important and welcome addition to the field of healthy nutrition and lifestyle medicine.

AdventHealthPress.com

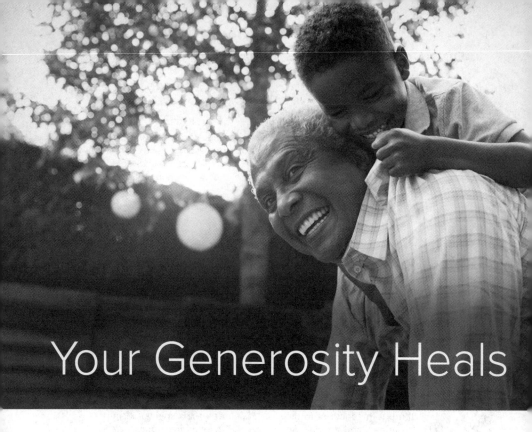

Your Generosity Heals

Generosity is powerful medicine. Studies show that when you give, it reduces stress, alleviates depression, and gives a greater sense of happiness to the giver. It may even lower your blood pressure and extend your life! *

When you give to **AdventHealth's Whole Person Health Education Fund**, you not only help yourself—you help create vital, innovative materials to educate and empower others. You help them discover the healthiest lifestyle on earth. A lifestyle that research shows will add years of health to the lives of those who embrace it.

100 percent of your gift will support these life-changing health resources. To learn more, or to make your Generosity Heals donation today, visit:

www.GenerosityHeals.Health

* See website for citations.